How To Pass
A Basic Arrhythmia Test with Ease

Arnel Carmona

Copyright © 2016 by Arnel Carmona
All rights reserved. This book or any portion thereof may not be reproduced or used in any manner whatsoever without the express written permission of the publisher except for the use of brief quotations.

Printed in the United States of America

First Printing, 2016

Preface

I had always been asked how to make ECG rhythms or arrhythmia reading easy. First of all it is not that easy. Second, what most textbooks will show are the easy or the "typical" ones. In the real world, maybe 10% of the time you will see complex rhythms. It is a different story if you will just ask me how to pass an ECG test. That is an easy one.

Most basic ECG tests will have basic and typical ECG strips. It will just basically show you one or 2 leads which could be lead II (with V lead). The length of the strip could be about 6 seconds or 10 seconds. There are only around 20+ rhythms to remember.

I hope you can use this material for a quick review for a basic ECG rhythm/arrhythmia test. All of the materials or ECG strips are from several years of sitting behind the telemetry monitor. So, this is the closest to the real thing you can see.

I hope you pass the pass the basic arrhythmia test with ease. Good luck!

Arnel Carmona

Contents

Understanding the ECG Paper 1

The Cardiac Conduction and the complexes 2

    Sinoatrial Node or Sinus Node 3

    Atrioventricular junction 3

    His Bundle Branch and the Purkinje fibers 3

The Electrodes and Leads 4

Five (5) Letters to Remember 6

Four (4) numbers to Remember: 2 intervals and 2 durations: 7

How to compute the rates 8

    Big box/square method 8

    Small box/square method 9

    Six (6) -second method 10

Sinoatrial Rhythms 11

    Sinus Rhythm 11

    Sinus Bradycardia 14

    Sinus Tachycardia 15

    Sinus Arrhythmia 16

        Phasic sinus arrhythmia 16

        Non-phasic sinus arrhythmia 17

        Ventriculophasic sinus arrhythmia 17

        Wandering Atrial Pacemaker 18

Multifocal Atrial Arrhythmia (MAA) - Multifocal Atrial Rhythm (MAR) and Multifocal Atrial Tachycardia (MAT) 19

Sinoatrial Block or Sinoatrial exit block 20

    SA block type I 20

    Second degree SA block type II 20

Sinus arrest/pause vs. Sinoatrial block 22

Premature Atrial Complexes 23

AV Junctional Rhythms 25

Atrioventricular Block (AV Block) 28

    First Degree AV Block 28

- Second Degree AV Block 30
  - Second degree AVB Type I (Mobitz I or Typical Wenckebach) 30
  - Second degree AVB Type I (Atypical Type I or Atypical Wenckebach)..............32
  - Second degree AVB Type II (Mobitz II) 33
  - Second degree AV block 2:1 AV conduction 34
  - Advanced/High-degree AV block..36
  - Third Degree AV Block 38
  - Paroxysmal AV block (ventricular standstill) 40

Atrial Flutter 41

Atrial Tachycardia 44

Atrial Fibrillation 45

Supraventricular Tachycardia..47

Ventricular Rhythms 51
  - Premature Ventricular Complexes (PVC) 51
  - Idioventricular Rhythm and accelerated idioventricular rhythm 53
  - Ventricular Tachycardia (VT) 54

Paced Rhythms 57

Review 60

References: 77

Index 79

Understanding the ECG Paper

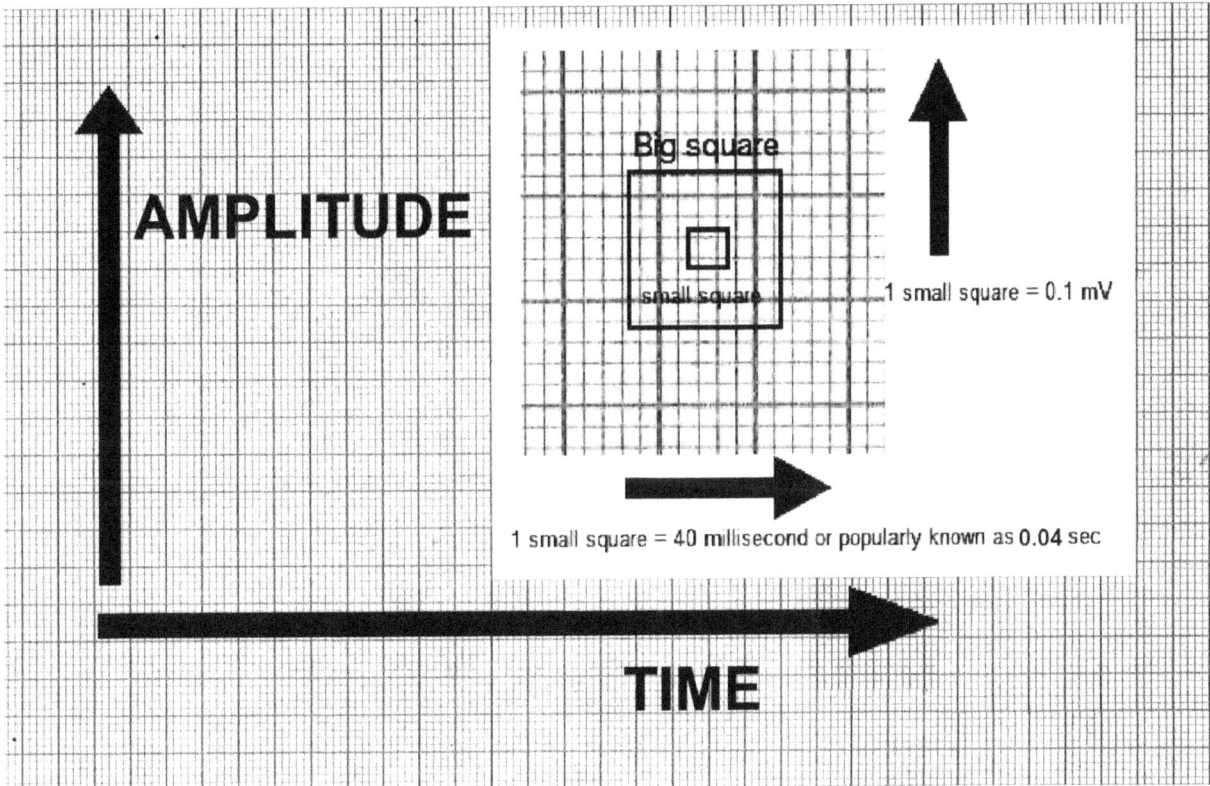

Figure 01 The ECG Paper

The ECG paper has small boxes and a big box which has a darker border. Inside the big box are 5 small boxes horizontally and vertically. The horizontal component tells time and vertical component tells the size or amplitude.

For time, **one small square is equivalent to 0.04 sec (s)** or 40milliseconds (ms). **One big box is equivalent to 0.20** sec (0.04 x 5 small squares). The durations of ECG complexes and intervals are calculated using these boxes

For the size of the complexes, one small square is equivalent to 0.1 millivolt (mV) or 1 mm. The size of complexes is used if there is hypertrophy and amplitude is also used for reference in ST elevations. In arrhythmia test, the size of the complexes is not our concern.

In basic ECG test, the typical setting is paper speed of 25mm/sec and 1x gain.

The Cardiac Conduction and the complexes

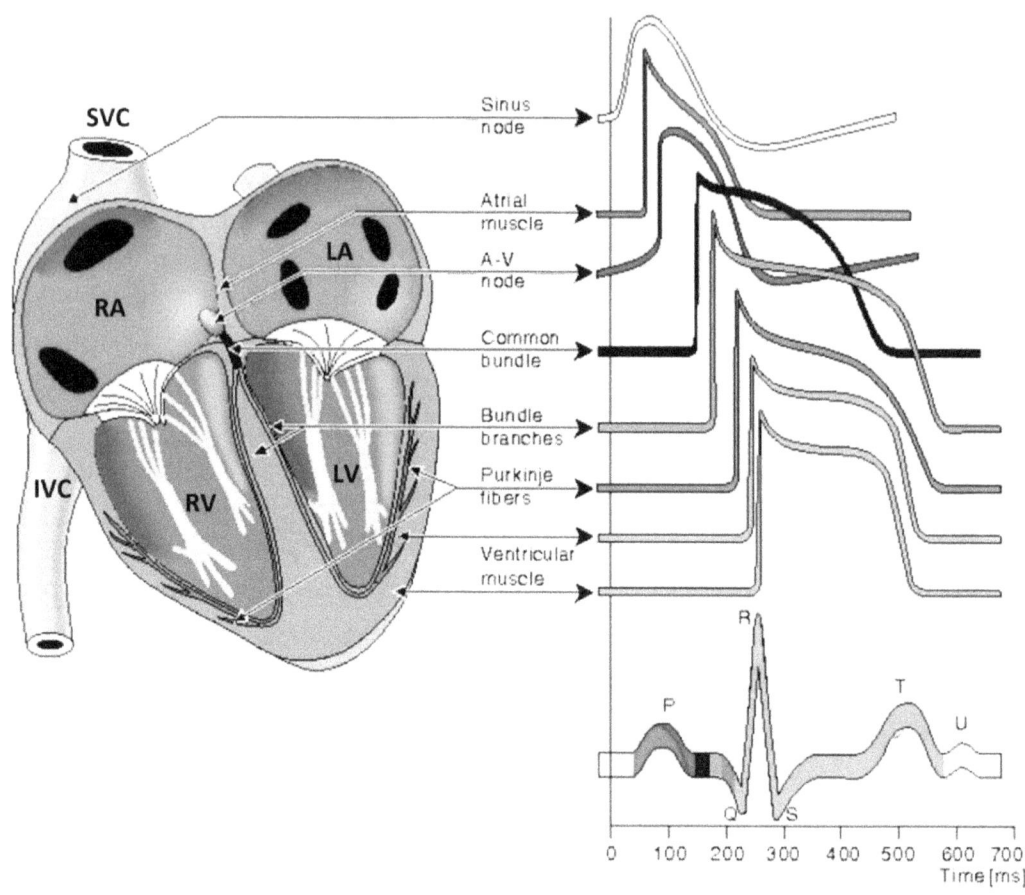

From: Jaakko Malmivuo & Robert Plonsey: Bioelectromagnetism - Principles and Applications of Bioelectric and Biomagnetic Fields, Oxford University Press, New York, 1995.

Figure 02 - The cardiac conduction system and the complexes. SVC - superior vena cava, IVC - inferior vena cava, RA - right atrium, LA - left atrium, RV - right ventricle, LV - left ventricle.

To make sense of an ECG these are the structures to remember:

Sinoatrial node (SAN)
Atrioventricular junction
Bundle branches
Purkinje fibers

Sinoatrial Node or Sinus Node

The *sinoatrial node* is located in the right atrium near the opening of the superior vena cava . This is a collection of specialized cells that is able to generate the *electrical signal* to initiate a heartbeat. The sinus node is the natural pacemaker of the human body. From here, the electrical signal spreads from the right atrium to the left atrium. This makes the right and left atria (atrium - singular) contract and pump blood to the ventricles (right and left ventricles). The electrical signal then reaches another special conducting tissue - the **AV junction**.

Atrioventricular junction

The AV junction (AVJ) is at the base of the wall dividing the atria or the interatrial septum. The AVJ is composed of the upper part, the **AV node** (AVN), and the lower part, the **bundle of His** (common bundle). The AVJ is the electrical connection of the atria and the ventricles. It is like a relay station. In the AV node, there is some delay in the electrical signal to allow the atrium to pump blood to ventricles and allow the ventricles to fill blood. The signal is then transmitted to the bundle of His which then divides into two branches the right and left bundle branch.

His Bundle Branch and the Purkinje fibers

There is one right bundle branch and two left bundle branches (left anterior fascicle and left posterior fascicle). The electrical signal reaches the ventricles via the **purkinje fibers**. The signal then spreads in the heart muscles (myocardium) going toward the outer part of the heart (endocardium).

These electrical currents are then recorded by the electrocardiogram (ECG) via **electrodes**.

The Electrodes and Leads

Simplistically, the direction of the cardiac electrical impulse is from the right upper part of the body going towards the left lower part of the body. To record this, stickers or electrodes (placed on the patient) attached to wires are connected to a machine or telemetry boxes. On the ECG machine or telemetry monitors this electrical signal is displayed as LEADS. These leads record the electrical voltage of the heart. The leads are like several individuals watching a baseball game. They are positioned at different areas of the stadium. In the case of the heart, the leads watch the direction of the electrical signal at different areas.

In routine telemetry, the six limb lead plus one or two chest leads are used. The **2 groups of limb leads are BIPOLAR limb leads (I, III and III) and AUGMENTED unipolar limb leads (aVR, aVL and aVF).** Because there are so much patients to be monitored, only 1 or 2 leads are used or displayed for arrhythmia monitoring.

The electrodes are attached to extremities (when doing 12-lead ECG) or on the body (Figure 03) for telemetry monitoring.

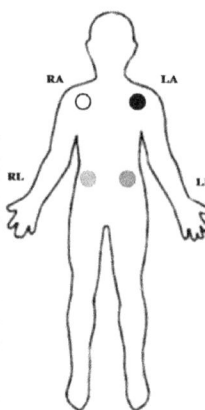

Figure 03 - Electrode placement on the body. It is color-coded.

In most ECG rhythm test or arrhythmia recognition test, lead II is used. Lead II records the voltage difference between the right arm (RA) and left leg (LL) with positive pole on the left leg. As a general rule, **an impulse going to the positive pole of a lead will create a positive or upright ECG deflection**. Lead II will generate a positive deflection (Figure 04) because the cardiac electrical impulse is moving from the right upper to the left lower part of the body (towards the positive pole of lead II). For aVR, the complexes are predominantly negative because the impulse is traveling away its positive pole.

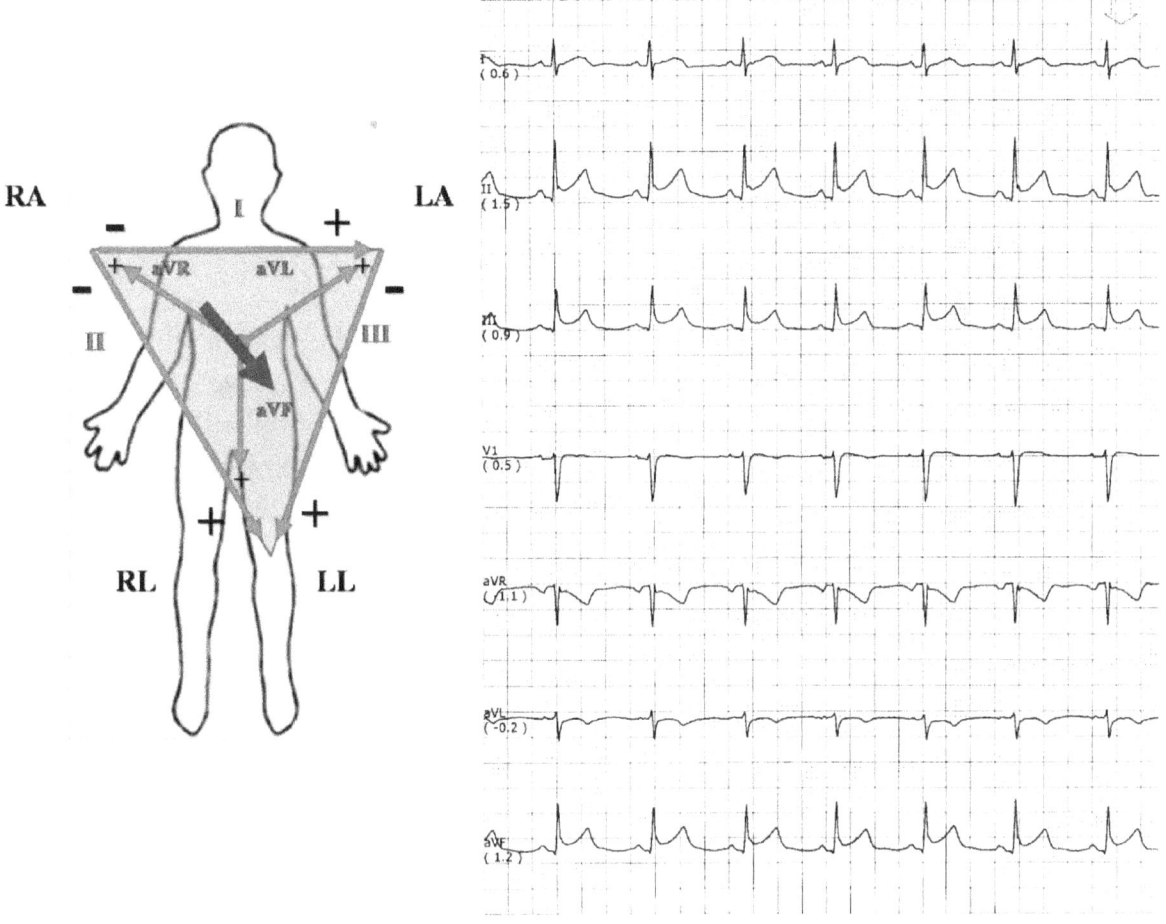

Figure 04- The different ECG leads and sample normal ECG tracing.

Five (5) Letters to Remember

There are only 5 letters that you need to learn or remember in ECG interpretation - P, QRS, T. Sometimes you see U waves.

To make it simple, let us use lead II. Starting from left to right there are 3 major deflections/complexes : **P, QRS and T waves**.

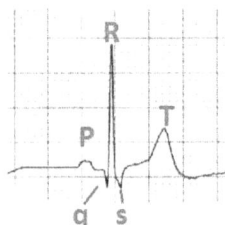

Figure 05 - The P, qRs and T complexes

- The P wave is atrial depolarization. This is the first small upright/positive wave seen.
- QRS complex is ventricular depolarization. The Q wave is the negative deflection. The R wave is the positive deflection and the S wave is the negative deflection. **For QRS complex nomenclature, capital letters are used to designate waves of larger amplitude and small letters are used to designate waves of smaller amplitude.**

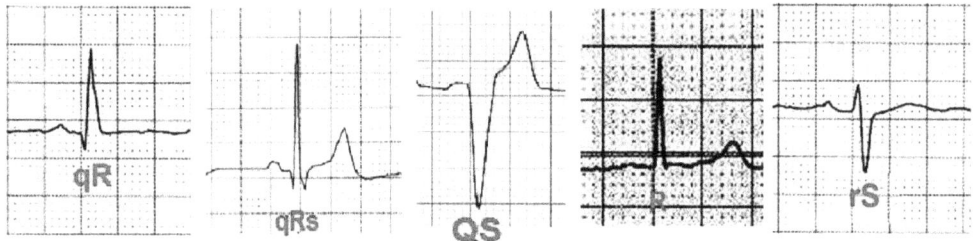

Figure 06 - QRS nomenclature

- T wave is the ventricular repolarization or recovery. This is the third upright wave.

Four (4) numbers to Remember: 2 intervals and 2 durations:

- *P wave duration* - The P wave duration is ≤ 0.11 sec and an amplitude of 2.5 mV. The P wave is generated from the sinoatrial node (SAN) which depolarizes in the direction from right to left atrium and superior to inferior. A longer P wave duration or tall P wave amplitude may mean atrial enlargement. This is a "nice to know" in ECG test.

- *PR interval (PRI)* - In adults, **the normal PRI is 0.12 - 0.20 sec (3 to 5 small squares)**. It is measured from the beginning of the P wave to the beginning of the QRS. Others would call this the "PQ interval" because it is the actual period being measured. The PRI represents the time required for the electrical impulse to advance from the atria, through the AV node, Bundle of His and Purkinje system (Figure 02). A prolonged PRI would **generally** be interpreted as **First Degree AV Block**.

- *QRS duration* - In adults, **the normal QRS duration is < 0.10 sec**. It is measured from the Q wave to the S wave. This is the ventricular activation or depolarization. **A wide QRS duration would mean a bundle branch block**, non-specific intraventricular delay (IVCD) or an aberrant beat. **In most ECG test, bundle branch block is an acceptable answer.**

- *QT interval* - It is measured from the Q wave to the end of the T wave. The largest T wave and with distinct termination is used. It is the duration of the ventricular electrical systole. QT interval is affected by the heart rate. So, a corrected QT (QTc) is computed. The most widely used formula is the Bazett's formula (QTc = QT interval / $\sqrt{RR}$). The upper limit for normal QTC is 470 ms in males and 480 ms in females. A QTc > 500 ms for both males and females is dangerous. A simple eyeball test for prolonged QTc is that, if the QT interval is more than 1/2 of the RR interval, then there is most likely a prolonged QTc. You can then use the formula. In most basic ECG test, you do not see strips with prolonged QTc.

In ECG test, just remember the normal PRI (0.12 - 0.20 sec) and QRS duration (< 0.10 sec).

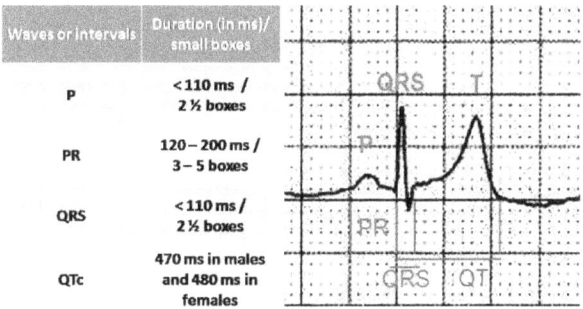

Figure 07 - The different ECG waves, normal durations and intervals

How to compute the rates

There are 3 ways to compute the rate:

- Big box/square method
- Small box/square method
- The 6-second Method

Big box/square method

The rate is computed by the RR interval for ventricular rate (or P to P for atrial rate) based on the big boxes it fit. A RR interval of 2 big boxes is equal to 150 bpm.

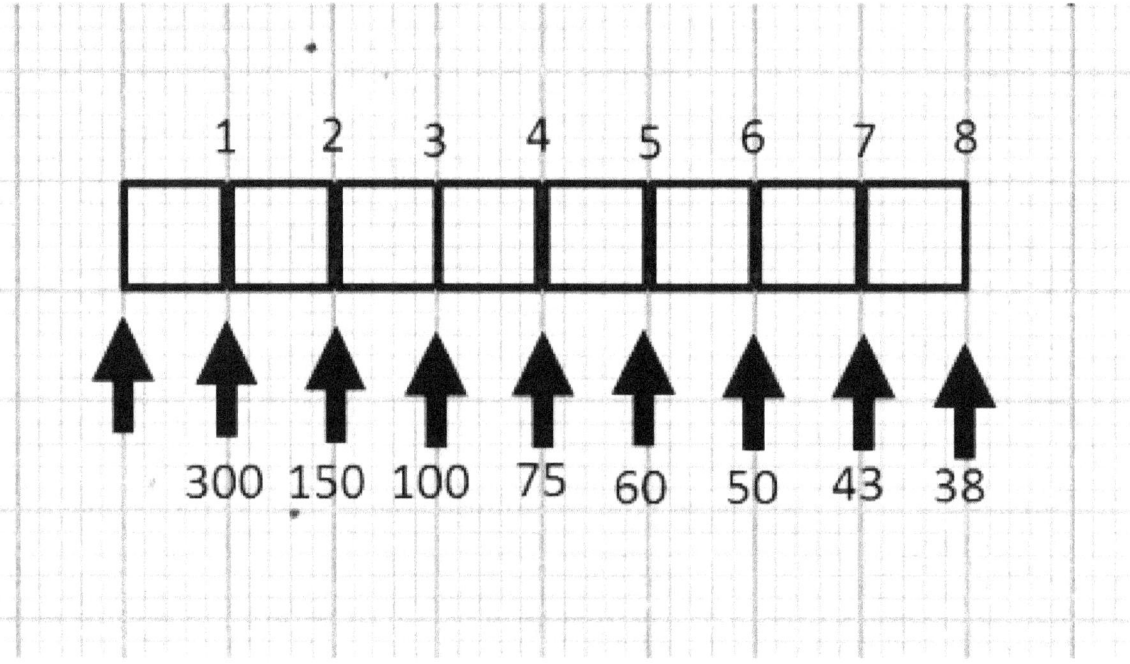

Figure 08 - The Big Box/square Method

Small box/square method
The number of small squares encompassing a RR interval is divided by 1500. So, in the example of 2 big squares will be 1500/10 = 150 bpm.

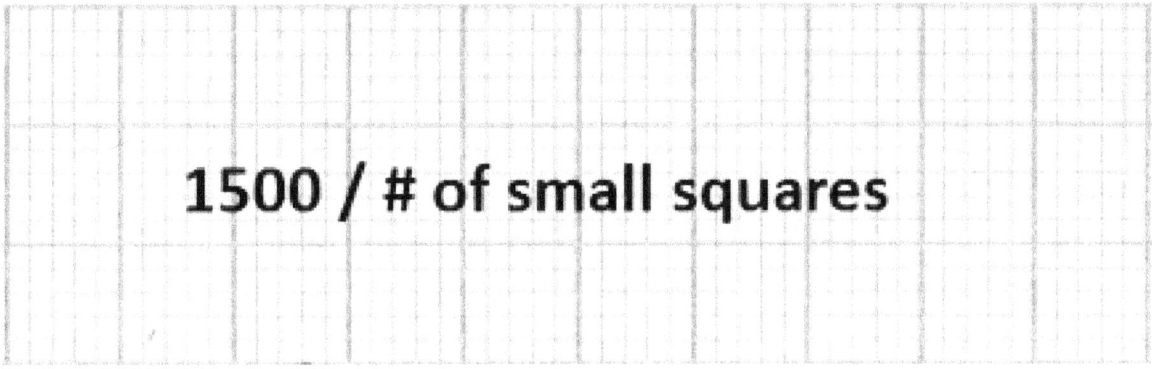

Figure 09 - The Small Box Method

Six (6) -second method

For irregular rhythms, the six-second method is very valuable. To get the rate, count the number of QRS complexes or R waves in a 6 second strip and multiply by 10. One small square or box is 0.04 sec (40 ms). One big box/square is 0.20 sec (200 ms). Five big boxes is 1 sec (1000 ms).

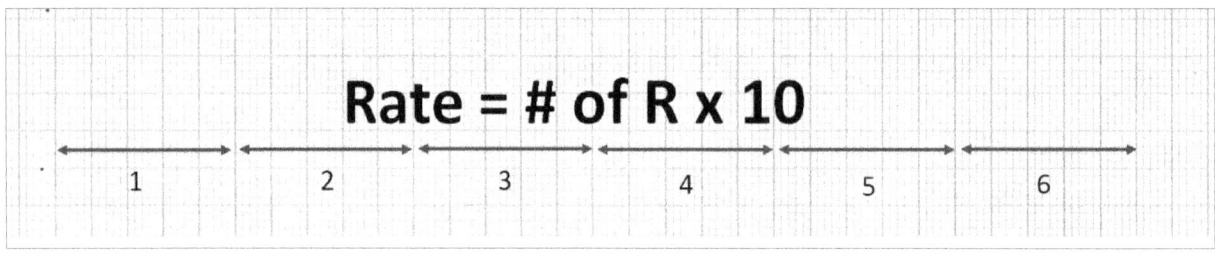

Figure 10 - The 6-second Method

In a telemetry strip, the 3 second is marked with small lines at the bottom (arrows). So, the rate below is about 13 x 10 = 130.

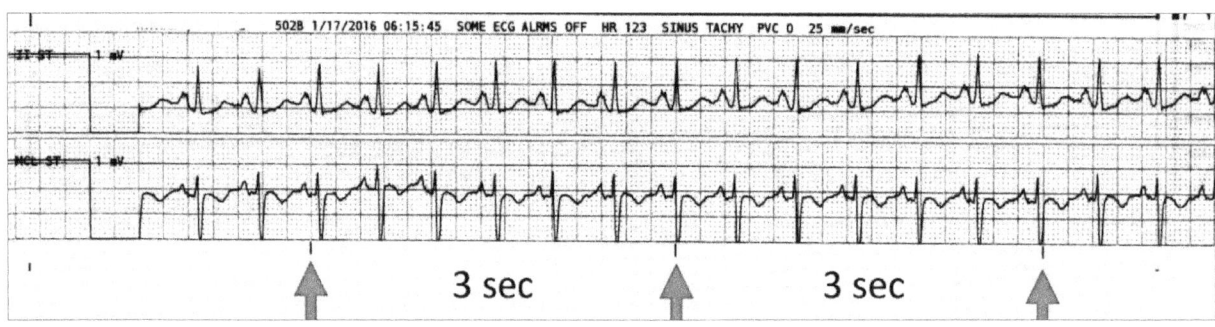

Figure 11 - *The 3 second marker is at the bottom of a printed strip*

Sinoatrial Rhythms

Sinus Rhythm

Normal sinus rhythm (NSR) is an impulse that originates in the sinus node (See Figure 02).

ECG Recognition:

It is recognized by the P wave morphology that is:

- **upright P in leads I, II and aVF**
- inverted in aVR
- variable in leads III and aVL
- upright in leads V4-V6 (in 12-lead ECG)
- most often biphasic (positive-negative) in leads V1 and V2
- with minor variations in morphology related to respiratory cycle

For ECG test taking purposes, an upright P in lead II is basically sinus rhythm.

PR interval (PRI) exceeds 120 ms or 0.12 s and can vary slightly with rate.

Rate can be between 60-100 beats/min. Most cardiologists agree that the operational limits for NSR range from 50-90 beats/min. Rates *lower than 60 beats/min* are considered to be (sinus) bradycardia and rates *higher than 100 beats/min* are considered to be (sinus) tachycardia.

***ECG TEST TIP** - During some atrioventricular blocks (AVB) which will be discussed later, the sinus P waves are not followed by a QRS. The atrial rate, which is computed by using the P to P interval, is higher than the ventricular rate. **The sinus rate (atrial rate in this case) is the basis for interpreting it sinus bradycardia or tachycardia**. So, you will see interpretations like sinus tachycardia with second degree AV block type II (with ventricular rates in the 50's) or sinus rhythm, complete heart block with idioventricular escape (with ventricular rate in the 30's).

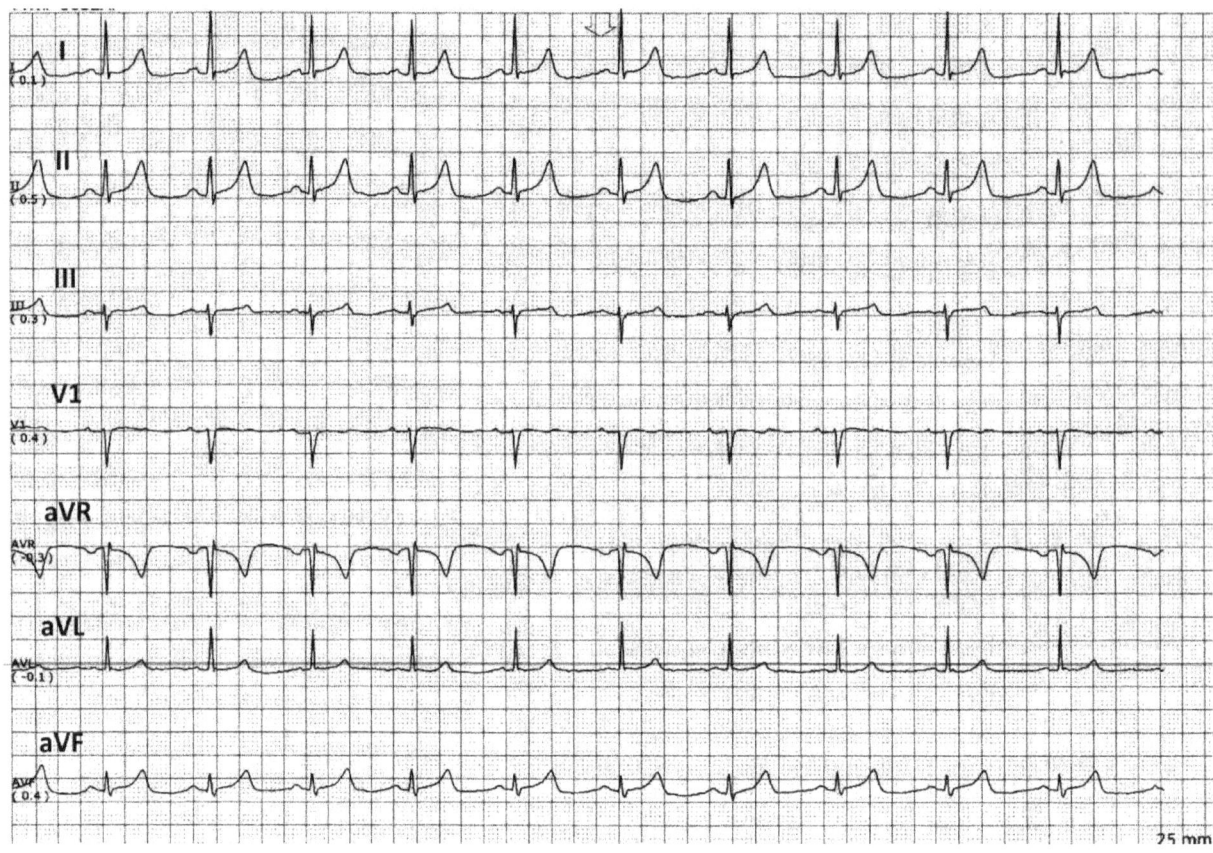

Figure 12 - Full disclosure view of a patient on telemetry. It shows all limb leads (I, II, III, aVR, aVL, aVF and V lead). The P wave has a sinus node morphology being upright in I, II and aVF and inverted in aVR. In ECG rhythm test, the lead/s commonly shown is lead II (and V1). So, so do not be overwhelmed with the 7-lead display.

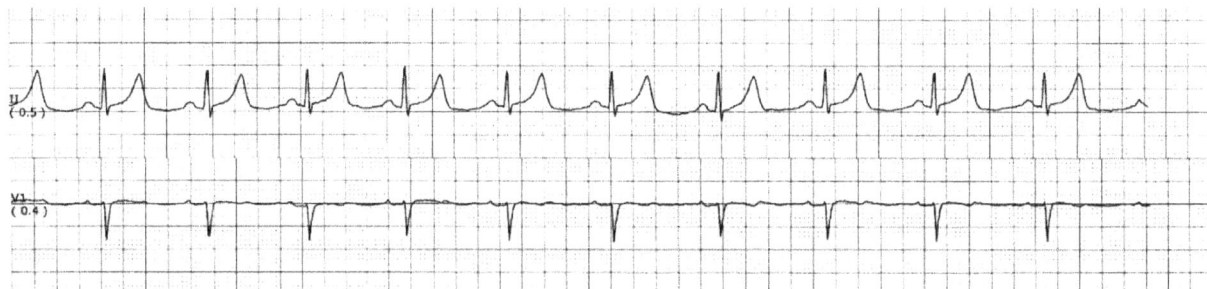

Figure 13 - **Normal sinus rhythm.** The 2-lead strips typically shown in ECG test showing sinus rhythm. **If you see an upright P wave in lead II like the one above with 1:1 P and QRS ratio, then generally the rhythm is sinus.**

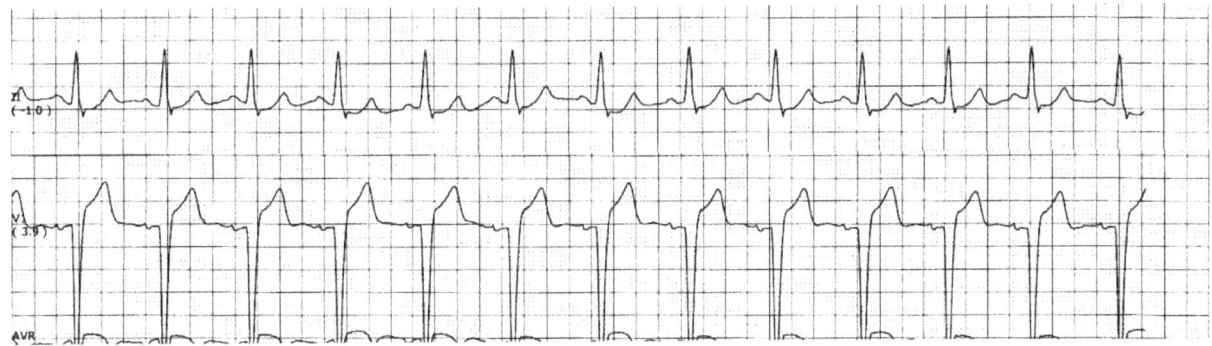

Figure 14- **Sinus rhythm with bundle branch block.** The P wave is upright in lead II followed by a wide QRS (0.12 sec) with QS pattern in V1 with a rate of about 75 bpm (4 big squares).

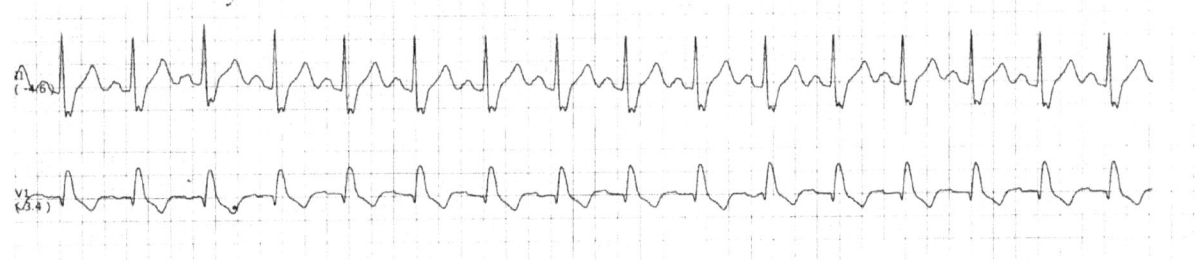

Figure 15 - **Sinus rhythm with bundle branch block.** The P wave is upright in lead II followed by a wide QRS with a qR pattern in V1 with a rate of about 93 bpm.

Nice to know

Bundle branch block can either be left bundle branch block (LBBB) or right bundle branch block (RBBB). There are certain criteria to make bundle branch block interpretation. However, generally, by looking at V1, if the QRS is predominantly negative then the block is most likely LBBB (Figure 14) and if the QRS is predominantly positive then the block is most likely RBBB (Figure 15). So, if you want to impress, you can interpret ECG strips as sinus rhythm with RBBB or LBBB. As mentioned before, bundle branch block is acceptable in basic arrhythmia test.

Sinus Bradycardia

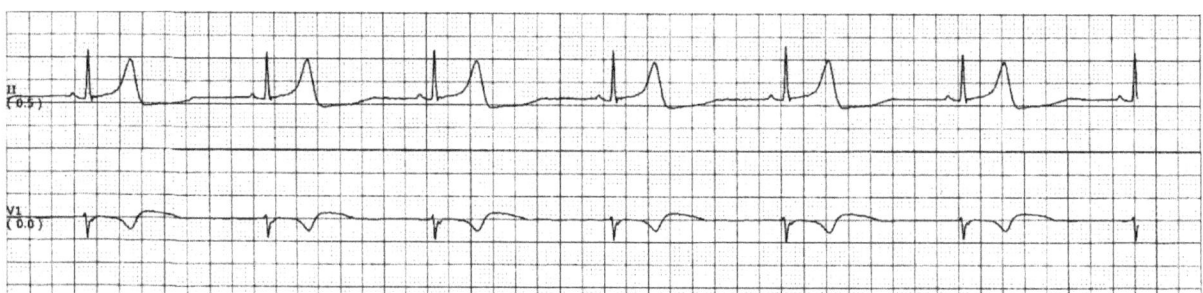

Figure 16 - **Sinus bradycardia.** This P wave is upright in lead II followed by narrow complex QRS with a PR interval of ~ 0.16 sec. The atrial and ventricular rates are about 38 beats per minute (bpm) or was computed by using the small box method of 1500 / 39 (small squares).

*ECG TEST TIP - For highly efficient reading or to make your life easier and save time during test, you can measure intervals and durations using a QRS that FALLS on a BIG BOX. In Figure 16, we can use QRS #5. You will notice that the QRS is exactly in line with a BIG BOX. From there we can measure the PRI (4 small squares or 0.16 sec), QRS duration (2 small squares or 0.08 sec and QT of about 12 small squares 0.48 sec (though you do not need this in basic arrhythmia test).

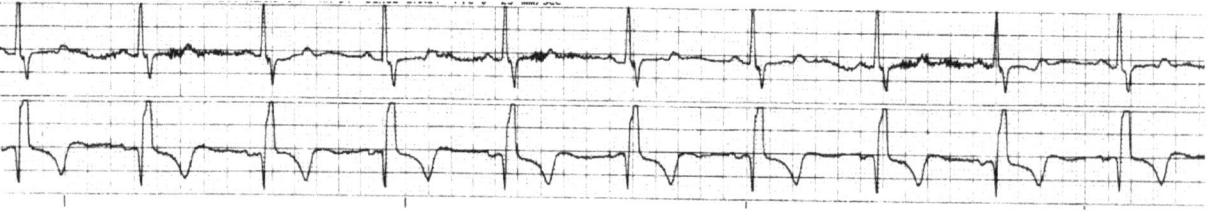

Figure 17 - **Sinus bradycardia with a bundle branch block.** This is lead II and V1. The P wave is upright in lead II followed by a wide QRS complex (QR pattern in V1) . The PR interval is 0.20 sec. There is one-to-one atrial to ventricular ratio at rate of about 56 bpm (1500/26 small squares).

Sinus Tachycardia

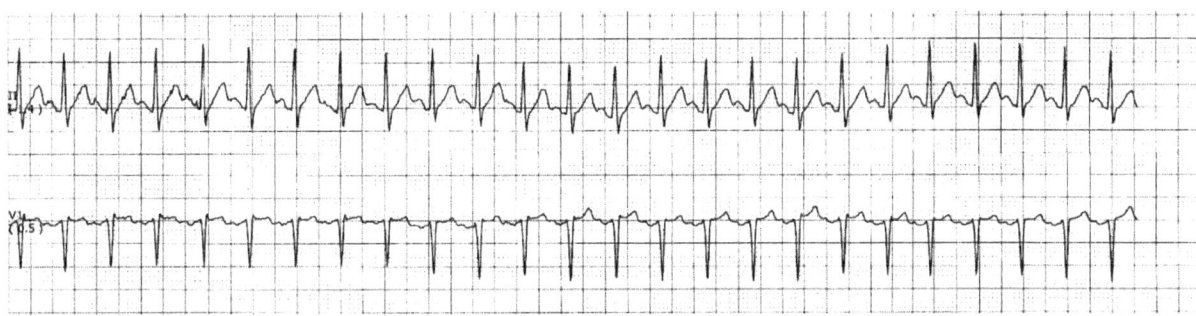

Figure 18 - **Sinus tachycardia.** The P wave is upright in lead II followed by a narrow QRS. The P wave here is seen right after the T wave. The rate is about 150 bpm.

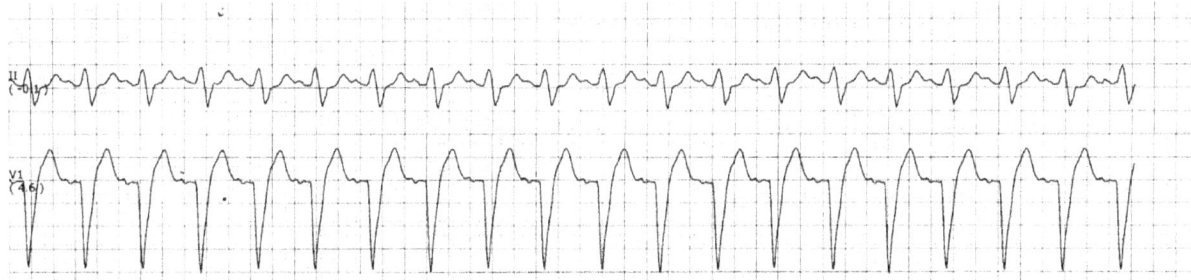

Figure 19 - **Sinus tachycardia with a bundle branch block.** The P wave is upright in lead II followed by wide QRS (QS pattern in V1). The P wave is wave is partly merged with the T wave. The rate is about 115 bpm.

Sinus Arrhythmia

ECG Recognition:

- The rhythm is irregular.
- The P wave and PR interval are normal
- The **P to P interval varies by 0.16 sec or 4 small squares.** So, strictly speaking, not all irregular sinus rhythm is sinus arrhythmia.

*ECG TEST TIP - Most basic ECG test would classify any irregular sinus rhythm as sinus arrhythmia. If you are taking the test in a computer and the rhythm is irregular with sinus P waves then choose sinus arrhythmia among the choices. If it is a paper test and it will be checked by a person and not a multiple choice test then you can argue if it is sinus arrhythmia or just sinus rhythm basing on the above criteria (P to P interval varies by 0.16 in sinus arrhythmia).

Nice to know:

There are 3 types: **phasic or respiratory, nonphasic or nonrespiratory and ventriculophasic sinus arrhythmia. However, in most ECG test sinus arrhythmia is acceptable.**

Phasic sinus arrhythmia

With phasic sinus arrhythmia, the rate is dependent on the respiratory cycle, increasing with respiration and decreasing with expiration. The pacemaker site in the sinoatrial node (SAN) shifts with respiration. The pacemaker site shifts higher the SAN, the heart rate and P wave amplitude or size in II, III and aVF increase. As the pacemaker shifts lower the SAN, the P wave amplitude and heart rate decrease. The heart rate changes gradually and rhythmically, thus differentiating it from non-phasic sinus arrhythmia.

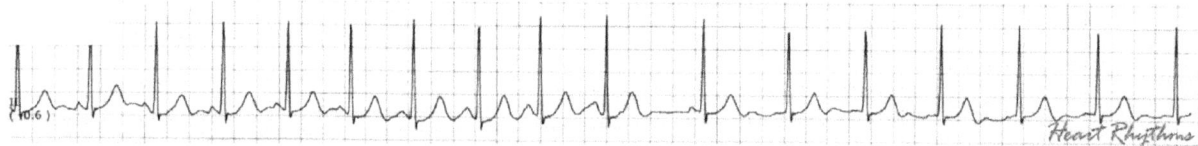

Figure 20 - **Phasic Sinus Arrhythmia.** The rhythm is irregular. The P wave is prominent at the beginning but there is a decrease in amplitude or size as the rate decreases.

Non-phasic sinus arrhythmia

For non-phasic (Non-respiratory) sinus arrhythmia , the P wave and PR interval are normal but the PP intervals vary at random and independent of any physiological function.

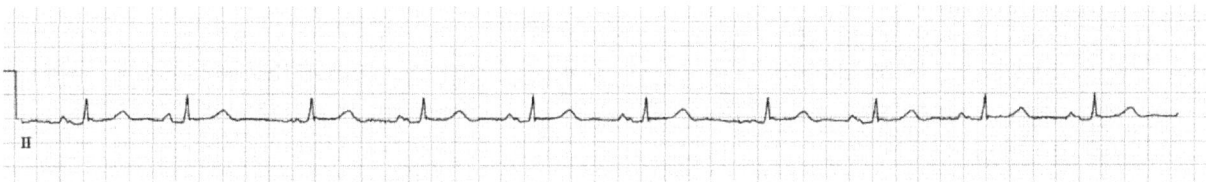

Figure 21 - **Non-phasic Sinus Arrhythmia.** The rhythm is irregular with upright P waves and normal PR interval. At a higher rate, the P wave is more prominent compared at slower rate.

Ventriculophasic sinus arrhythmia

For ventriculophasic sinus arrhythmia , the P to P interval encompassing a QRS complex are shorter than the intervals without an intervening QRS complex. Ventriculophasic sinus arrhythmia is noted in the presence of AV block.

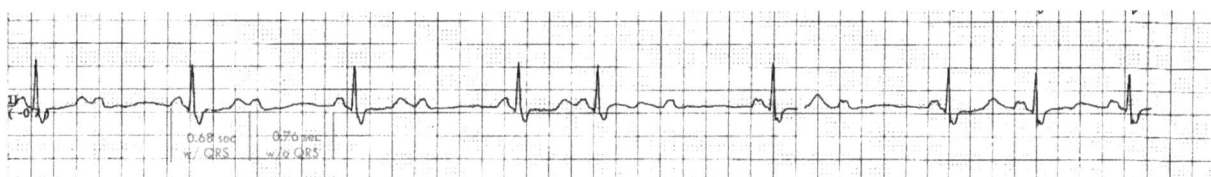

Figure 22 - **Ventriculophasic sinus arrhythmia.** The rhythm is still sinus because there are upright P waves seen in lead II. The atrial rate about 88 bpm with second degree AV block type II (Mobitz II) manifesting as 2:1 and 3:2 AV conduction (AV block is discussed later). **The P to P interval encompassing a QRS is shorter compared to that without an intervening QRS complex (0.68 s vs 0.76 s).** This is a *"nice to know "* in most ECG test.

Wandering Atrial Pacemaker

WAP is a variant of sinus arrhythmia. There is passive transfer of dominant pacemaker focus from the sinus node to latent pacemakers. **The change (in P wave shape) occurs gradually.** There is only one pacemaker that is in control.

ECG Recognition:

The change in P wave contour is gradual and after several cycles the pacemaker shifts back to the sinus node. Do not confuse WAP with multifocal atrial rhythm (MAR) which is discussed later.

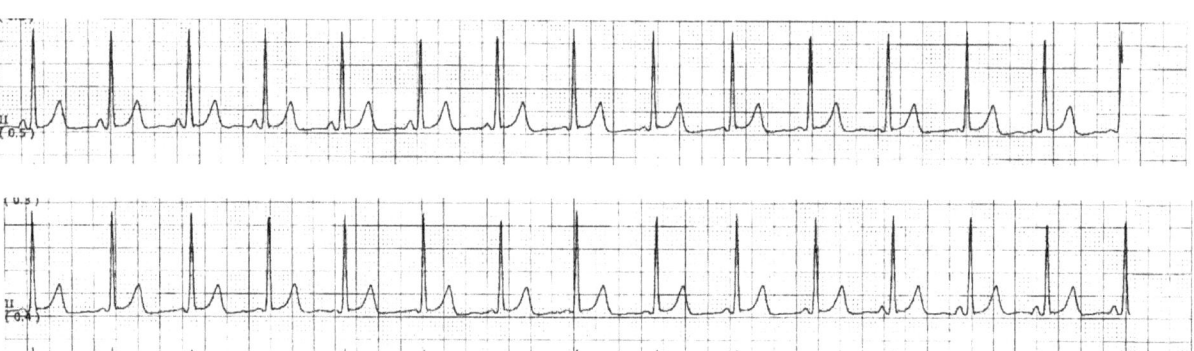

Figure 23 - **Wandering Atrial Pacemaker.** These 2 strips are 10 seconds long lead II strips that are seconds apart that were intentionally printed to illustrate gradual change of P wave contour/morphology.

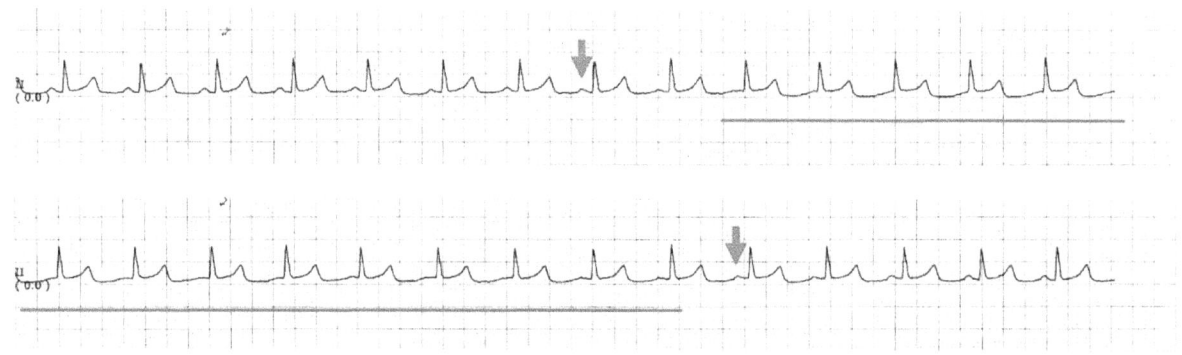

Figure 24 - **Wandering Atrial Pacemaker .** Long lead II strips of one patient taken at different time intervals to highlight the gradual disappearance of distinct P wave (upper strip) and gradual appearance of distinct P wave (lower strip).

*****ECG TEST TIP**: You may not see WAP on a test because a long strip is needed to show transition of P wave shape or morphology.

Multifocal Atrial Arrhythmia (MAA) - Multifocal Atrial Rhythm (MAR) and Multifocal Atrial Tachycardia (MAT)

ECG Recognition:

- **Variable P-wave morphology of at least 3 different configurations.**
- **Irregular PP, RR and PR intervals.**
- The change in P wave morphology is not gradual in contrast to WAP.
- The rate is **less than 100 bpm for multifocal atrial rhythm (MAR).** If the rate is **more than 100 bpm, the rhythm is called multifocal atrial tachycardia (MAT) or chaotic atrial tachycardia.**
- **Another name for MAR is multifocal PAC.**
- Some of the conducted P waves are wide because one of the bundle branches is still in refractory period. The electrical impulse is blocked on one of the bundle branches. This delay the cardiac conduction. Thereby creating a wide QRS. This intermittent block is called aberrancy.

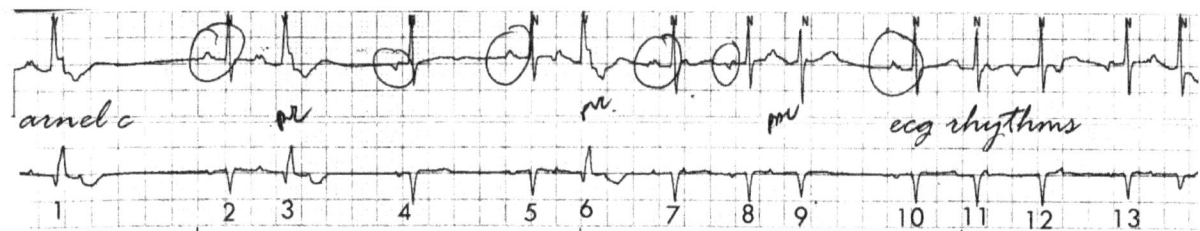

Figure 25 - **Multifocal atrial rhythm (MAR)/ multifocal atrial tachycardia (MAT).** This is an irregularly irregular rhythm with multiple P wave morphologies. The PP, RR and PRI varies. The rate varies from 60 to 150 bpm.

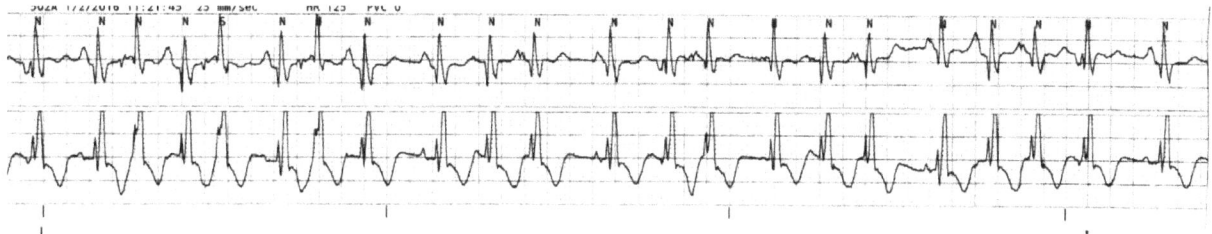

Figure 26 - **Multifocal Atrial Tachycardia with a bundle branch block.** This is an irregularly, irregular rhythm with several different P wave morphology and variable PR interval. The QRS is wide (~0.12 sec). The rate is about 120-130 bpm using the six-second method.

*ECG TEST TIP - Most likely you will not see this in a test. If this would appear, most would call Figure 25 as wandering atrial pacemaker. However, the irregularity of the pattern eliminates WAP as the ECG interpretation. Also, in WAP the change in P wave change is gradual.

Sinoatrial Block or Sinoatrial exit block

Nice to know:

Sinoatrial blocks (also called SA exit block or sinoatrial exit block) result when there is an abnormality in the conduction from the SA node to the surrounding atrium. As with AV block, SA block is characterized as first-, second-, and third-degree, with second-degree blocks subclassified as type I and type II.

First-degree SA block represents an increased time for the SA node's impulse to reach and depolarize the rest of the atrium to form a P wave. It cannot be seen on the surface ECG because the impulse generation in the SA node do not produce a deflection.

Second-degree SA block can be seen on the surface ECG. It could either be type I or type II.

ECG Recognition:

SA block type I

- There is progressive increase in the interval for each SA nodal impulse to depolarize the atrium and create a P wave until an SA nodal impulse does not depolarize the atrium at all.

- On the surface ECG, there is gradual shortening of the P-P interval with an eventual "dropped" P-QRST complex

- There is "group-beating" or may manifest as irregular sinus rhythm with pauses.

Second degree SA block type II

- there is a "dropped" P-QRST complex with the P-P interval surrounding the pause that is two to four time the length of the baseline P-P interval. This is because there is a consistent interval between the SA node impulse and the depolarization of the atrium until the SA nodal impulse is not conducted.

Third degree SA block occurs when none of the sinus impulse failed to depolarize the atrium. This will appear as junctional rhythm with no P waves.

*ECG TEST TIP - You will not encounter SA block in most basic ECG test but if it does then you are ready for this.

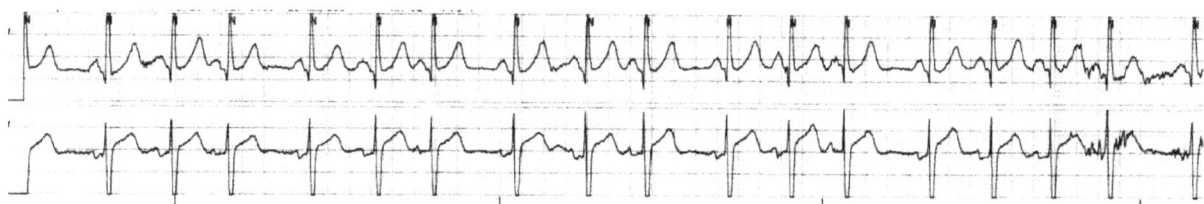

Figure 27 - **Second degree SA block type I or sinoatrial exit block type I.** There is group-beating (3 QRS in a group). There is shortening of the PP interval until the missing P QRs complex.

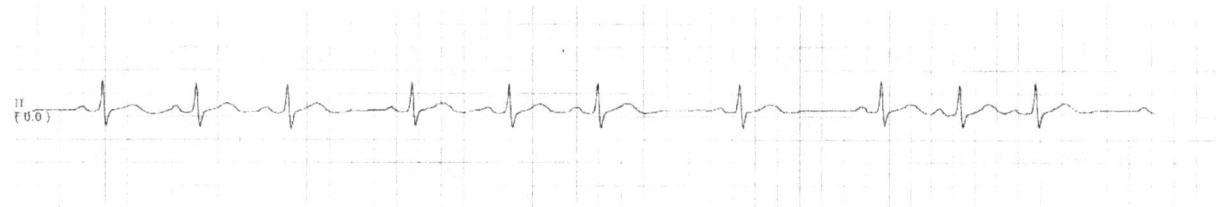

Figure 28 - **Sinoatrial exit block type I.** There is group beating and shortening of the PP interval until there is a dropped PQRST. There is no evidence of a PAC on all the leads that can explain the sudden bradycardia.

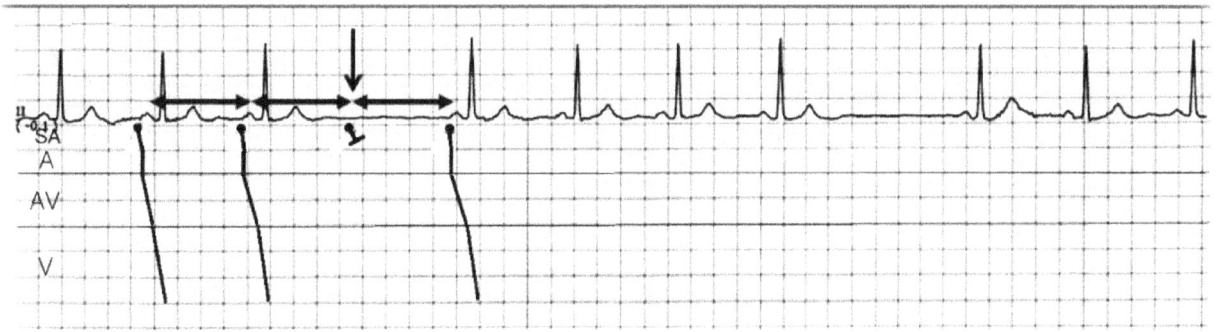

Figure 29 - **Second degree SA block type II.** The surrounding PP interval around the pause is equal to 2x the baseline PP interval. In short, the expected PQRST complex did not show up.

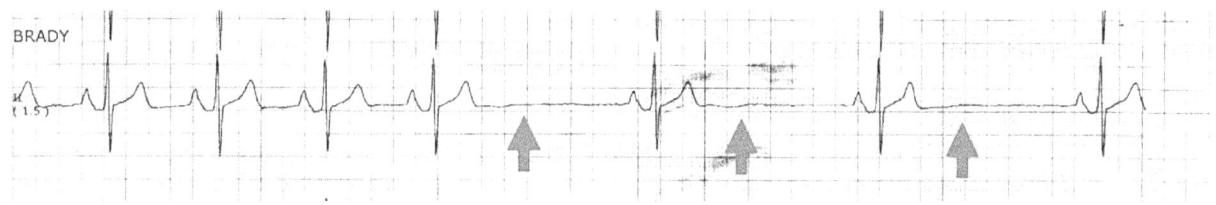

Figure 30 - **Sinoatrial exit block type II.** There is the complete absence of the expected PQRST. The surrounding pause is equal to 2x the baseline PP interval.

Sinus arrest/pause vs. Sinoatrial block

Sinus pause refers to brief failure while sinus arrest refers to a prolonged failure of the SA node. There is no universally accepted definition to differentiate the two. This is due to the failure of the SA node to generate an impulse.

On the surface ECG, it is seen as absence of PQRST complex. To differentiate it from SA block is to measure the **PP interval**. During <u>**sinus pause, the PP interval is not a multiple of the baseline PP interval**</u> while **SA block** should be a **multiple of the baseline PP interval**.

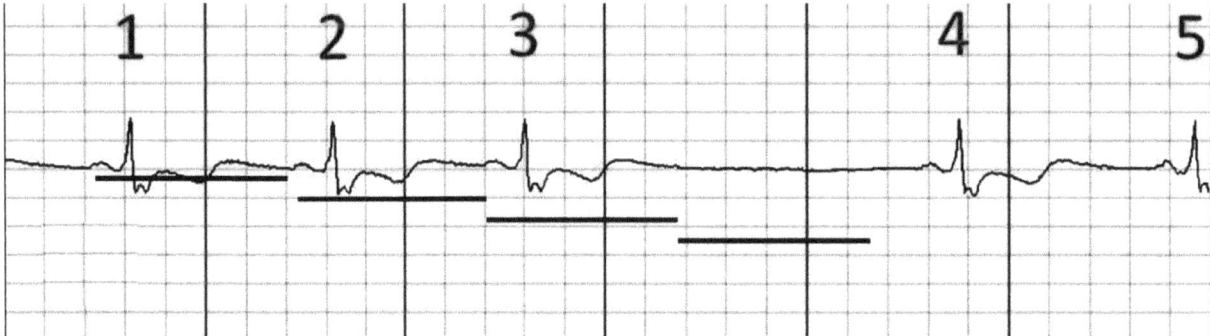

Figure 31 - **Sinus pause/arrest**. This is sinus bradycardia (~57 bpm) with a bundle branch block. The pause is not equal to the baseline PP interval making sinoatrial exit block type II unlikely.

Premature Atrial Complexes

ECG Recognition:

- <u>**The ECG feature of a premature atrial complex (PAC) is prematurity and altered P wave morphology.**</u>
- The closer its origin to the SA node, the more it will look like the sinus P wave. A PAC originating in the low atrium will have a low amplitude or inverted P wave in II, III and aVF.
- <u>**A PAC will have a PRI more than 0.12 s compared to premature junctional complex (PJC) which will be 0.12 s or less.**</u>
- PAC can manifest as a complex that appears after every other normal beat (bigeminal pattern); after 2 normal beat or the PAC is the 3rd beat (trigeminy; etc.)
- However, *some PJC's will have delayed retrograde conduction*. So, it suggested to call complexes with inverted P wave morphologies **AV junctional rhythms**.

There are 3 fates of a PAC: conducted with normal QRS morphology, conducted with aberrancy and a PAC that is not conducted. Depending on the degree of prematurity, a PAC will be conducted to the ventricles with normal of long PRI. A PAC that falls during the absolute refractory period of the AV node will not conduct (non-conducted PAC). A PAC that conducts through the AV node but finds the right bundle branch refractory will conduct with a RBBB morphology (conducted with aberrancy). Refractory period is the time when an excitable tissue is not responsive to an incoming stimulus.

- PAC conducted with normal QRS duration
- PAC conducted with aberrancy
- Non-conducted PAC

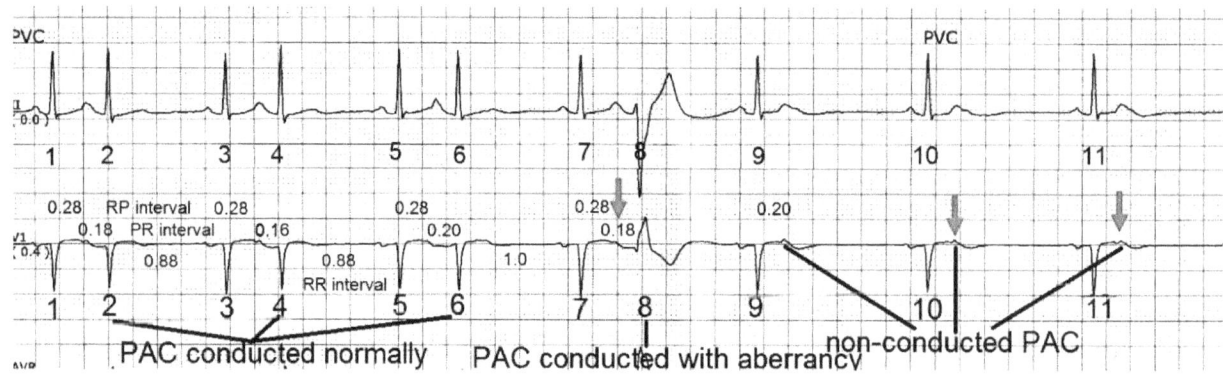

Figure 32 - **Sinus rhythm with PAC in bigeminy conducted normally, conducted with aberrancy and blocked or non-conducted PAC.** Every other beat is PAC or in bigeminal pattern. The first 3 PAC's which created QRS # 2,4 and 6 are conducted with a normal QRS morphology. The 4th PAC which is which created QRS #8 is conducted with a right bundle branch block (RBBB) configuration. The last 3 PAC's which are after QRS #s 9,10 and 11 are not conducted.

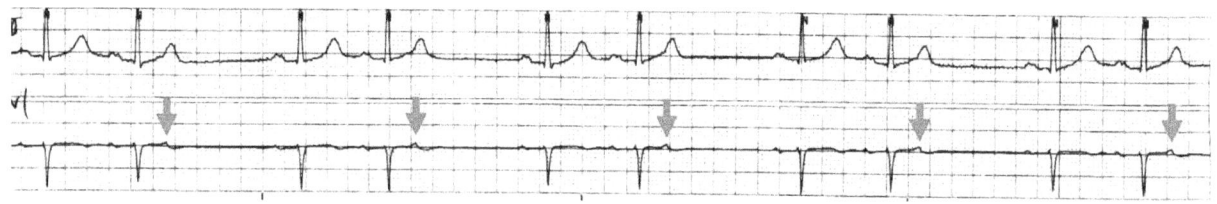

Figure 33 - **Sinus rhythm with PAC in trigeminy that is blocked or non-conducted.** This is a challenging ECG. The non-conducted P wave is better seen in V1 as a small distortion of the T wave on the second QRS (arrows). To determine that this is a P wave on top of a T wave, compare the shape of previous T wave. The second T wave is more prominent. Thus, we can prove that this is indeed a P wave that is premature that is not conducted.

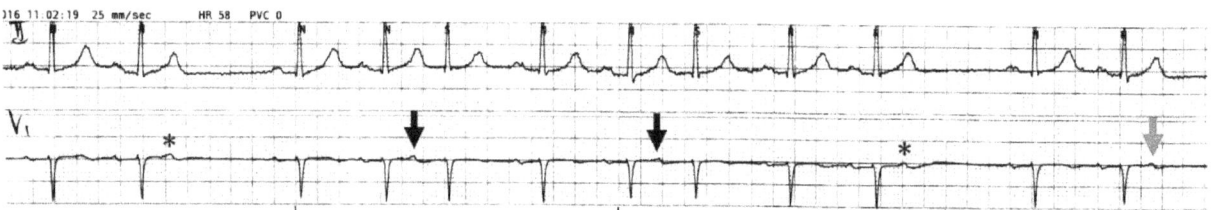

Figure 34 - **Sinus rhythm with PAC in trigeminy (non-conducted and conducted with normal QRS).** This is another challenging ECG. The PAC's are better seen in V1. The PAC with asterisk are not conducted while the PAC with arrows are conducted with a normal QRS but with a prolonged PR interval. The reason of the prolonged PRI on the conducted PAC is because the AV node is in a relative refractory period. It will allow AV conduction but it will delay the AV conduction because it is still recovering from the previous sinus impulse.

AV Junctional Rhythms

ECG Recognition:

A junctional impulse depolarizing both the atria and ventricles is characterized by:

- **Negative or inverted P wave in II, III and aVF, upright in aVR and isoelectric in I**
- **The negative P wave can be seen before or after the QRS.**
- **P wave is not seen if both the atria and ventricles are activated simultaneously because the P wave is buried in the QRS.**
- In the absence of AV conduction abnormality, the PRI and RP interval is approximately 0.12 and 0.19 sec, respectively.
- An isolated inverted P wave may be seen if it failed to conduct to the ventricles
- QRS may be normal in the absence of a bundle branch block or aberration.
- **Junctional rhythm rate varies from 40-60 bpm (may be as low as 30).**
- **Accelerated junctional rhythm is between 60-100 bpm.**
- **Junctional tachycardia rate is above 100 bpm.**

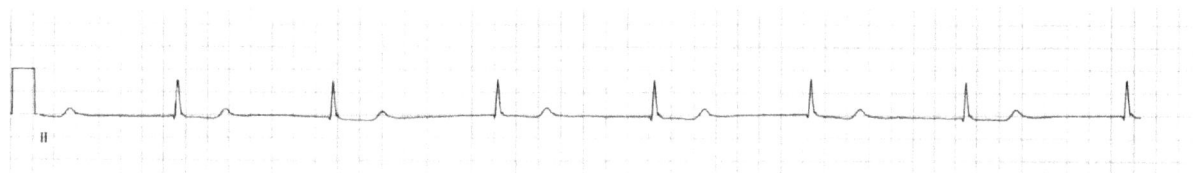

Figure 35 - **Junctional Rhythm** - This is a regular narrow QRS complex rhythm with no distinct P waves at a rate of about 43 bpm (1500/35 small squares).

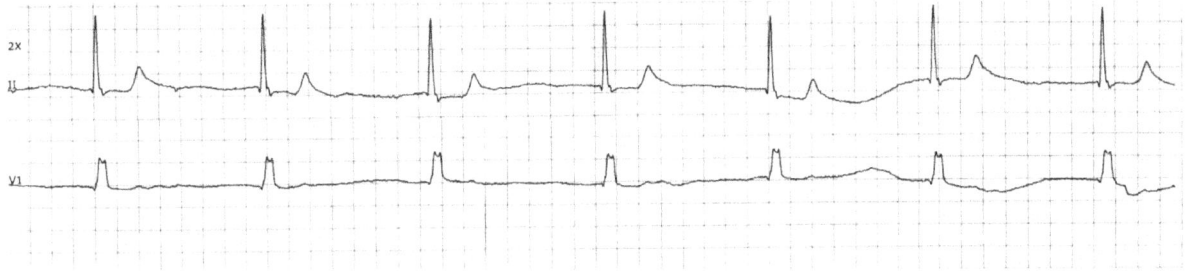

Figure 36 - **Junctional Rhythm with a bundle branch block.** This is regular wide QRS complex rhythm with no distinct P waves at a rate of about 38 bpm (1500/39 small squares). If this was a ventricular rhythm, the T wave should be opposite the direction of the R wave in lead II. Thus, it is possible to have a junctional rhythm with a bundle branch block.

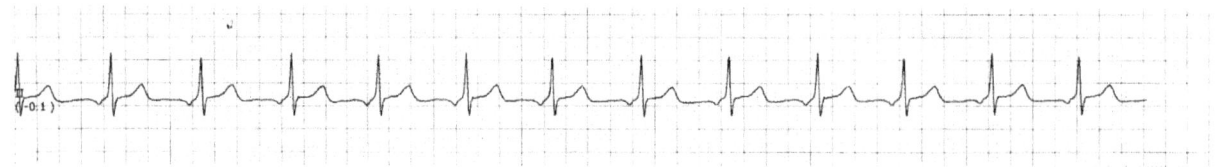

Figure 37 - **Accelerated Junctional Rhythm** - This is a regular narrow QRS complex rhythm with an inverted P wave before the QRS with PRI of about 0.12 sec. The rate is about 75 bpm.

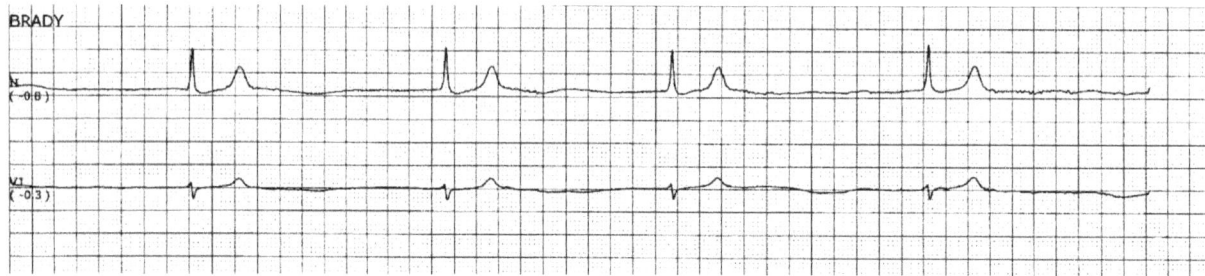

Figure 38 - **Junctional rhythm.** This is a regular narrow QRS complex rhythm with no P waves seen. The rate is about 25 bpm. The rate is computed using the 6-second method (1500/58 = 26 bpm).

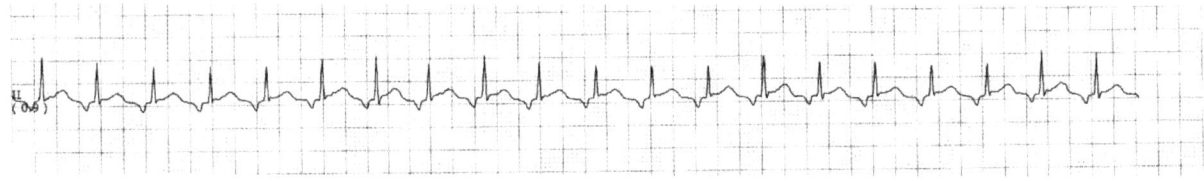

Figure 39 - **Junctional Tachycardia.** This is a regular narrow QRS complex tachycardia with an inverted P wave before the QRS with a PRI of about 0.08 sec.

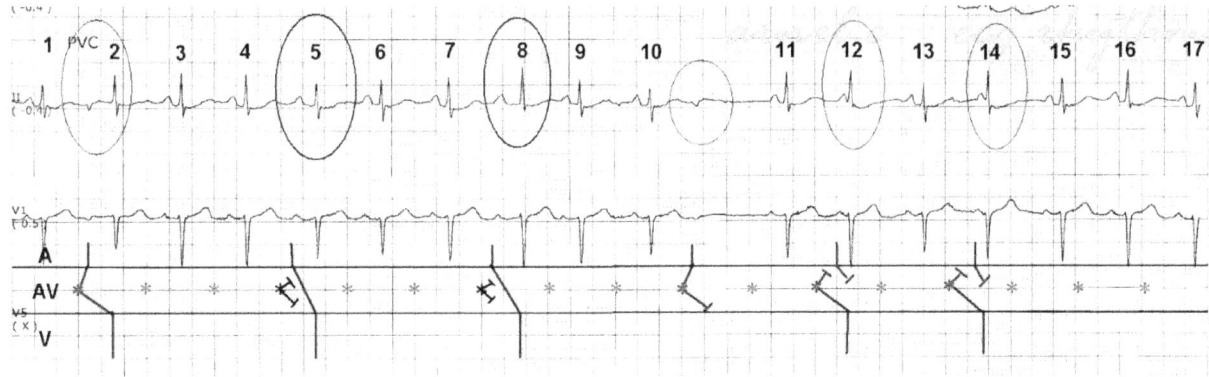

Figure 40 - Most likely you will not see this in basic ECG test. This strip is just shown to highlight what "tricks" junctional beats can do to surface ECG. Remember that a junctional beat cannot be seen on the ECG. It is seen only when it manifest as an inverted P wave or a QRS with no P wave. In this challenging ECG strip, in QRS #2, the PRI is about 0.20 sec or there is delayed conduction from the junction to the atrium. In QRS # 5 and 8, the P wave is upright but the PRI is longer compared to the other QRS complexes. This is because the AV junction is in the relative refractory period. The junction allowed conduction from the incoming sinus beat but it delayed or slowed down the conduction. So, there is a prolonged PRI. The junctional beat after QRS #10 is not conducted to the ventricles but conducted to the atrium as manifested by an inverted P wave. This is because the AV junction is refractory to any incoming impulse. In QRS # 12 and 14, the PRI is very short. This is because the atrium is depolarized by a sinus impulse while the AVJ junction depolarized the ventricles.

Atrioventricular Block (AV Block)

In AV block, conduction is altered between the atrium and the ventricles. It may manifest as prolonged PR interval, a dropped P waves or a P waves without a QRS after it.

First Degree AV Block

ECG Recognition:

- First degree AV block manifest with a **PR interval greater than 0.20 sec that remains constant.**
- The P wave is normal in morphology.
- The QRS is normal in duration or the wide if there is an existing bundle branch block.

The lengthening of the PRI is due to the conduction delay in the atrium, AV node, or the His-Purkinje system.

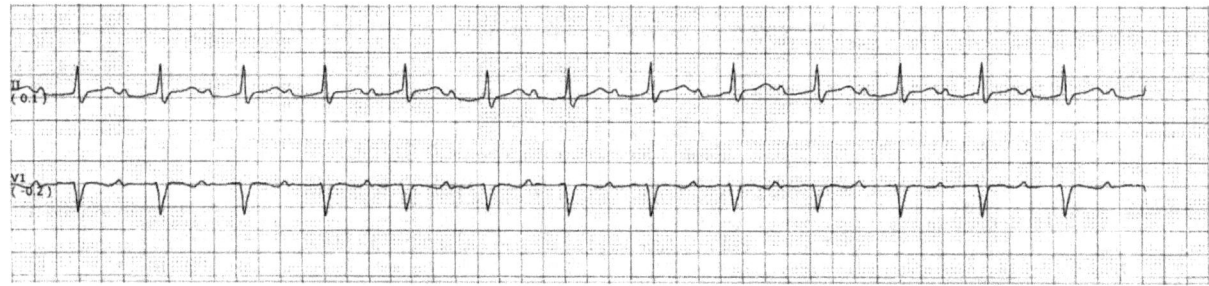

Figure 41 - **First degree AV block.** The rhythm is sinus at about 83 bpm. The PRI is prolonged at 0.36 sec (9 small squares).

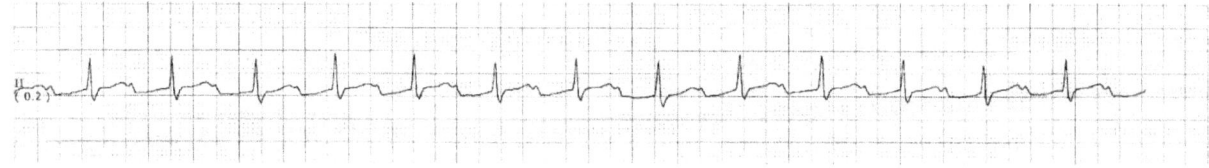

Figure 42 - **First degree AV block.** The PRI at about 0.40 sec (10 small squares) and the P wave is seen merging with the T wave.

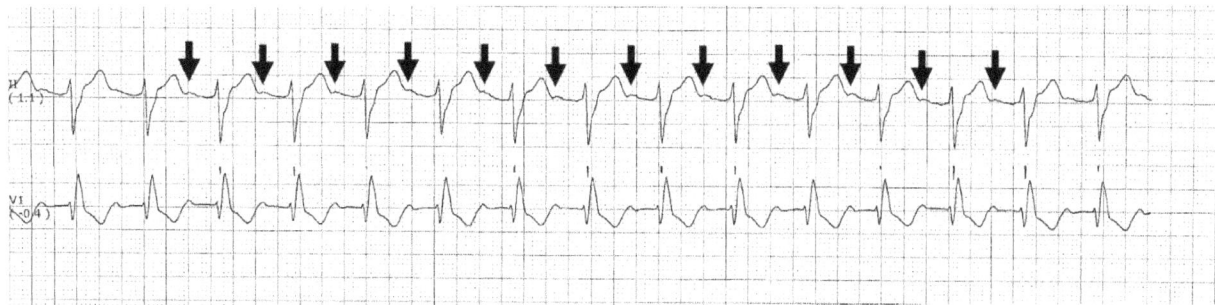

Figure 43 - **Sinus rhythm, first degree AV block with bundle branch block.** This is a regular wide QRS rhythm (0.14 sec) with prolonged PRI (~0.26 sec). The P waves (arrows) are seen right after the T waves and looked flat.

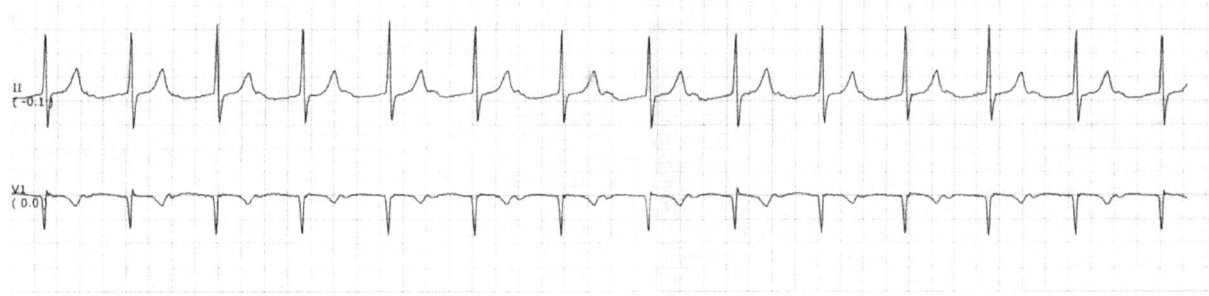

Figure 44 - **Sinus rhythm, first degree AV block (long PRI).** This is regular narrow QRS rhythm with a rate of about 80 bpm with a PRI of about .40 sec.

Second Degree AV Block

Second degree AVB Type I (Mobitz I or Typical Wenckebach)

ECG Recognition (Typical Type I):

- Second degree AV block type I is characterized by a normal P wave.
- **The PRI progressively lengthens until a P wave is not followed by a QRS.**
- As the PRI lengthens, there is shortening of the RR interval.
- The RR interval containing the dropped P wave is less than 2x of the shortest RR interval.
- The PRI (may be normal or prolonged) of the first conducted P wave is shorter than the last conducted PRI.
- The largest increment in the PRI is usually on the second conducted P wave.
- There is "group-beating" on the ECG.

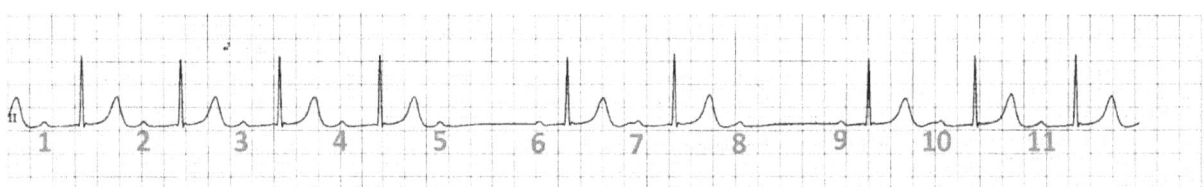

Figure 45 - **Sinus rhythm, first degree AV block, second degree AV block type I.** There is a regular sinus P wave at a rate of about 68 bpm. There are 2 non-conducted P waves (P waves # 5 and 8).

The middle ECG strip shows sinus rhythm with narrow QRS. The first conducted P (#6) wave has a prolonged PRI (~0.24 sec). The second conducted PRI (#7) is 0.36 sec (9 small squares). This is followed by a non-conducted P wave (#8). P wave # 9 has a PRI of 0.24 sec.

*ECG TEST TIP: The easiest or fastest way to determine if this is second degree AV block type I or type II is to compare the PRI around the non-conducted P wave. In type I, the PRI before the non-conducted P wave is longer than the PRI after the non-conducted P wave. In this case, if we look at the P wave # 5, the PRI is 0.36 s (9 small squares) vs 0.24 s (6 small squares). Try comparing the PRI around the non-conducted P wave # 8.

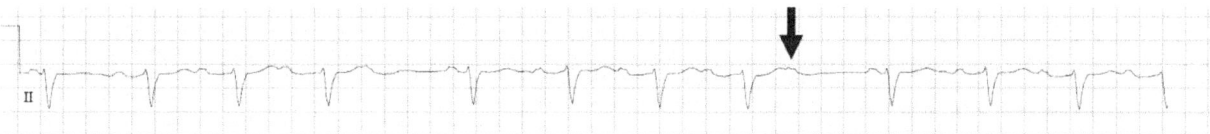

Figure 46 - **Sinus rhythm, second degree AV block type I, bundle branch block.** There is a regular sinus P wave at a rate of about 75 bpm (1500/20 small squares). Focusing on the middle of the ECG strip, There is a non-conducted P wave that is "sitting" or on top of the T wave. You have to use a caliper to march the P wave up to that point. The second clue that there is a P wave on top of that T wave is the distorted shape of the T wave. Having determined that there is non-conducted P wave, you can then compare the PRI surrounding that non-conducted P wave. In this case, it is 0.28 sec vs .16 sec.

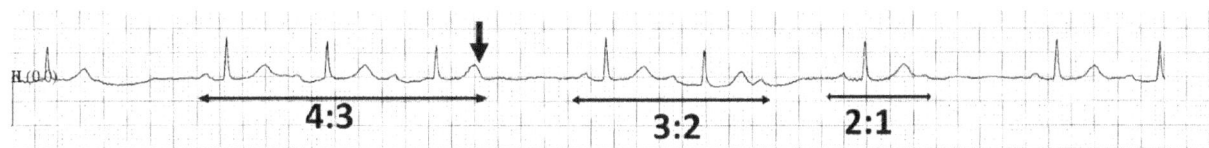

Figure 47 - **Sinus rhythm with second degree AV block type I.** There is regular sinus P wave at a rate of about 75 bpm. Another way of looking Type I second degree AV block is the "group-beating" it creates. In this ECG strip, there is a group of 3, 2 and 1QRS complexes. This is because of the ratio created by 4:3, 3:2 and 2:1 which means that there are 4 P waves and 3 QRS and 3 P waves and 2 QRS complexes and 2 P waves and 1 QRS. In the 4:3 group, the dropped or non-conducted P wave is "buried" in the T wave (arrow). You can also label this as sinus rhythm with 4:3, 3:2 and 2:1 AV Wenckebach.

Nice to Know

Second degree AVB Type I (Atypical Type I or Atypical Wenckebach)
ECG Recognition (Atypical Wenckebach):

- When the conduction ration exceeds 6:5 (6P and 5 QRS) or 7:6, the PR interval increment becomes unpredictable.
- The PRI may remain the same (prolonged), then increase, and then the dropped beat.

You may not see this in basic ECG test.

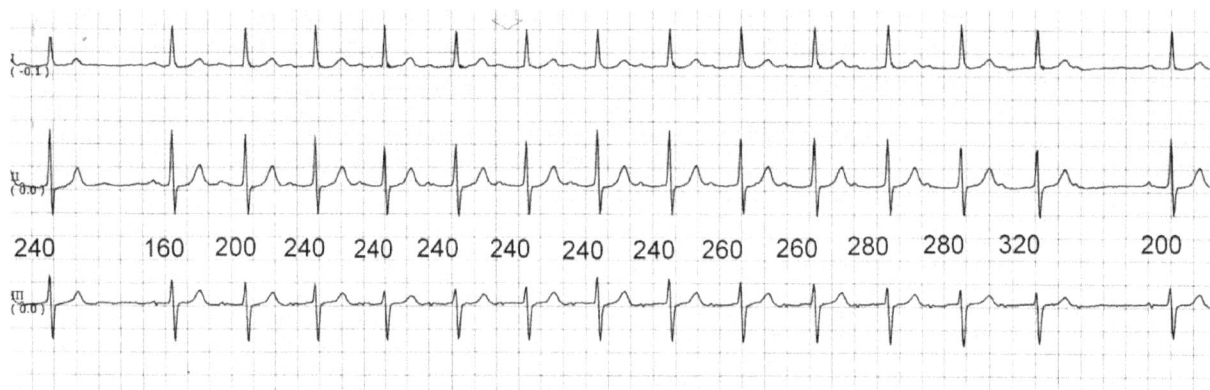

Figure 48 - **Sinus rhythm with atypical Wenckebach** - There is progression in PRI prolongation but at times the PRI remained the same and then increased. So, the increment becomes unpredictable. The number is the PR interval measured in millisecond.

Second degree AVB Type II (Mobitz II)
ECG Recognition:

- There is **constant PR interval (normal or prolonged) before a P wave is dropped**.
- The QRS is usually widened because the location of the block is often infranodal.
- The QRS complex maybe narrow indicating a more proximal location of the block (AV node).

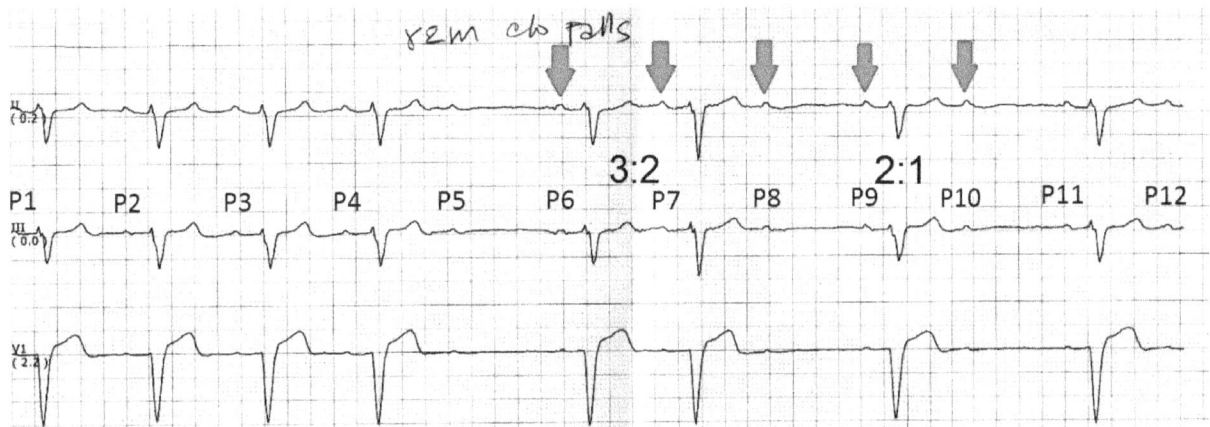

Figure 49 - **Sinus rhythm, first degree AV block, second degree AV block type II, bundle branch block.** There is regular sinus P wave at a rate of about 65 bpm. P waves # 5,8 and 10 are not conducted. The PRI surrounding the non-conducted P waves are the same. The baseline PRI is prolonged (~.24 sec). There is also a wide QRS (0.12 sec). This patient was admitted due to a fall. The patient eventually got a pacemaker.

*ECG TEST TIP: As mentioned before, the fastest way to differentiate second degree AV block type I from type II is to compare the PRI surrounding the dropped or non-conducted P wave. In type II, The PRI surrounding the dropped or non-conducted P wave is the same.

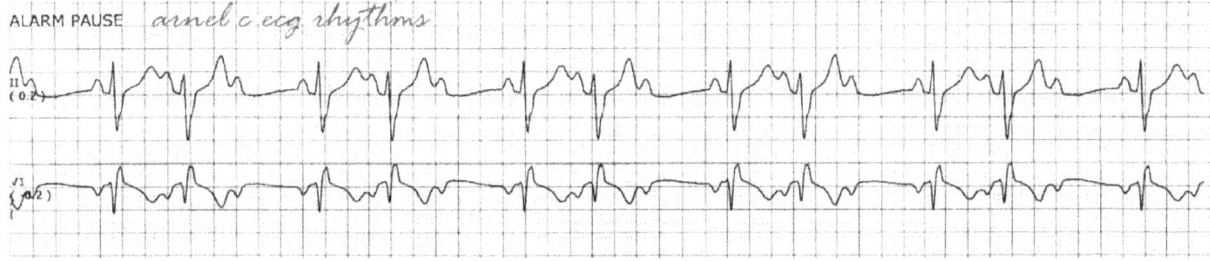

Figure 50 - **Sinus rhythm, second degree AV block type II, bundle branch block.** There is a regular sinus P wave at a rate of about 100 bpm with a PRI of 0.16 sec and a wide QRS. Every third P wave is not conducted. The PRI surrounding the non-conducted P wave is the same (0.16 sec). This can also be called **second degree AV block type II with 3:2 AV conduction** (3 P : 2 QRS).

Second degree AV block 2:1 AV conduction

ECG Recognition:

- During sinus rhythm, 2 to 1 AV block manifest as 2 P waves followed by 1 QRS.
- **This is a subtype of second degree AV block.**
- A 2:1 AV block could either be second degree AV block type I or type II.
- **A long strip is needed to capture the mechanism or true nature of a 2:1 AV block.**

*ECG TEST TIP: In most ECG test, this is labeled as second degree AV block. However, this rhythm should/must be labeled as second degree AV block 2:1.

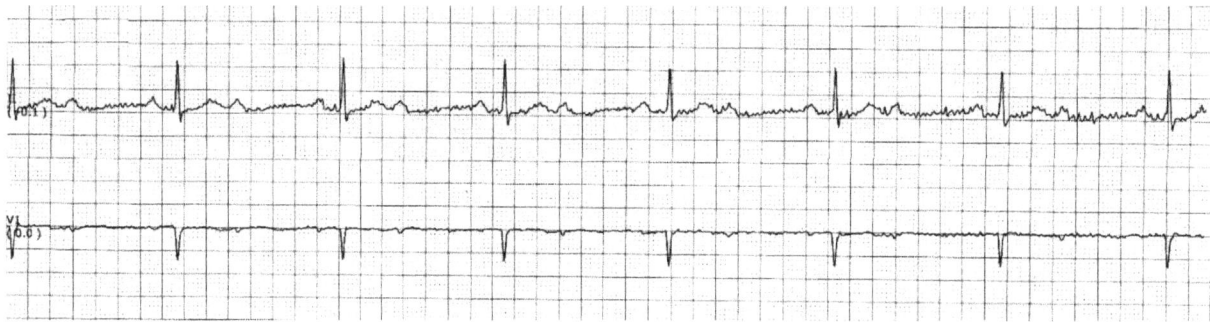

Figure 51 - **Sinus rhythm, first degree AV block with second degree AV block 2:1.** There is a regular sinus P wave at a rate of about 88 bpm. Every other P wave is not conducted or in a 2:1 pattern. There is prolonged PRI (0.24 sec) and normal QRS duration.

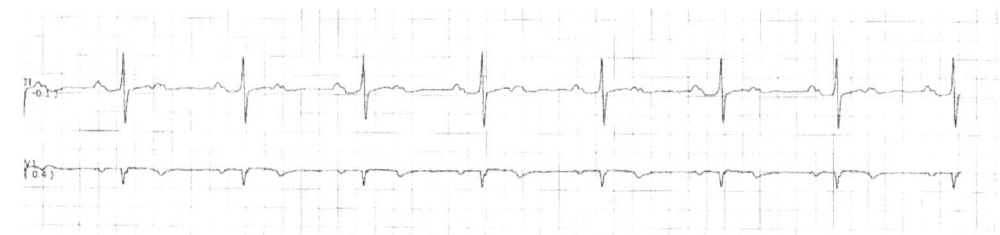

Figure 52 - **Sinus rhythm, first degree AV block, second degree AVB 2 to 1**. There is a regular sinus P wave at a rate of about 94 bpm with a narrow QRS complexes. Every other P wave is conducted or with a 2:1 pattern.

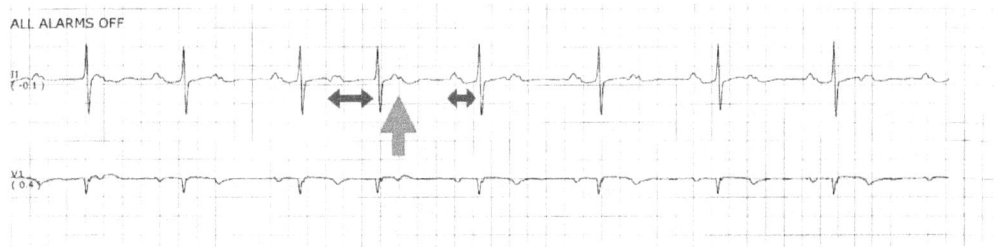

Figure 53 - The previous 2:1 rhythm is revealed on this strips as due to second degree AV block type I. Unlike in static ECG where you randomly capture the cardiac activity, in telemetry settings you can review the saved strips and know the true nature of the arrhythmia. In this strip, there is gradual prolongation of the PRI then the dropped beat (red arrow). So, this case is **second degree AV block 2:1 due to Wenckebach (type I) mechanism.**

Advanced/High-degree AV block
ECG Recognition:

- During sinus rhythm, when 2 or more P waves are not conducted the term given is advanced or high-grade AV block.
- The QRS may be wide or narrow.
- This is a clinically concerning **variant of Mobitz II** and often implies advanced conduction disease and may progress to complete heart block.

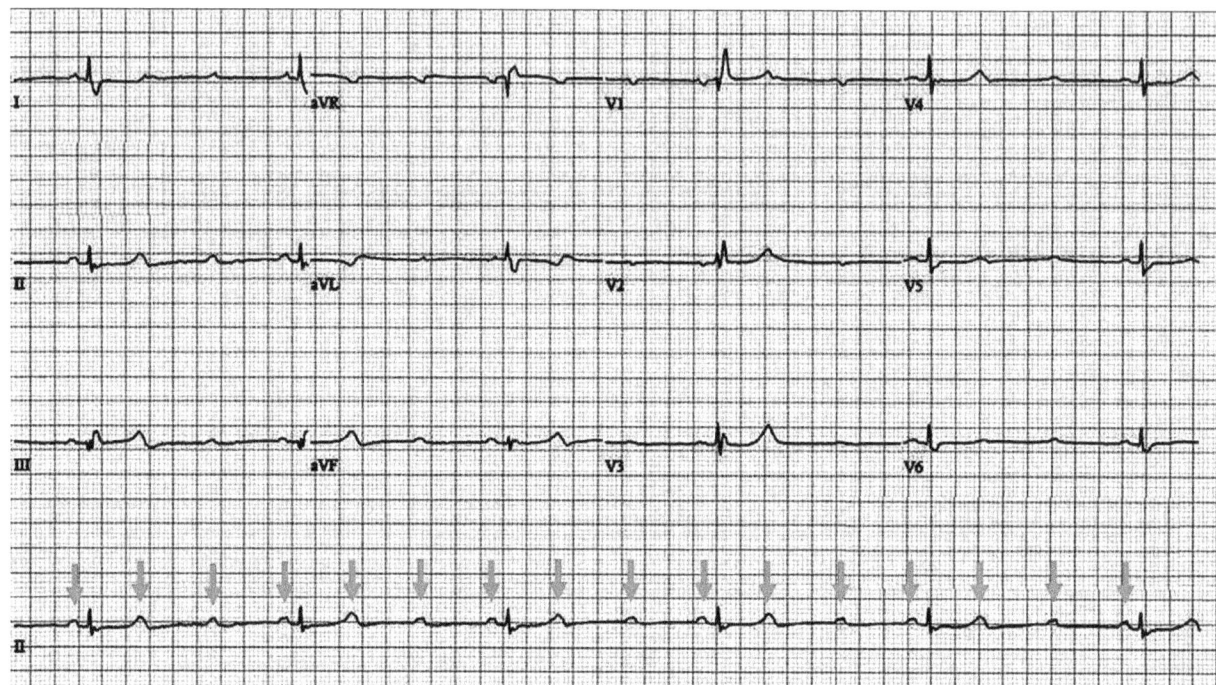

Figure 54 - **Sinus rhythm, advanced or high-degree AV block, right bundle branch block.** There is a regular sinus P wave at a rate of ~100bpm and a wide QRS with a qR pattern in V1 indicating right bundle branch block with a rate of ~33 bpm (1500/45 small squares). Some of the P waves are "buried" in the QRS or hidden from view. A caliper is needed to march-out the P wave. For every 3 P waves, there is 1 QRS or there is 3:1 pattern of conduction.

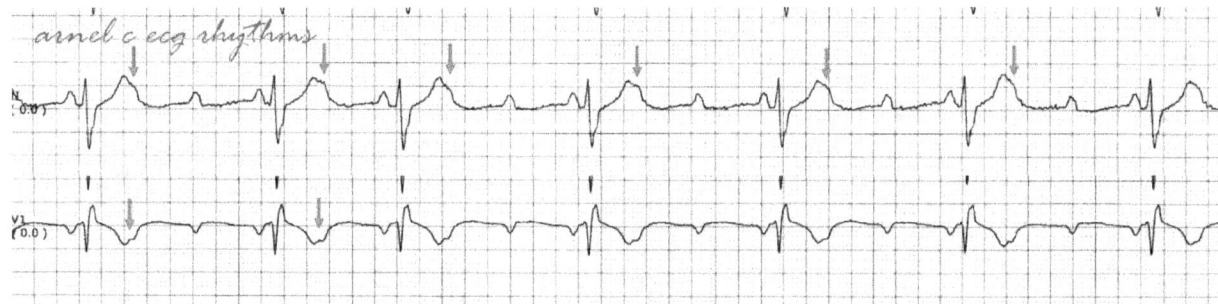

Figure 55 - **Sinus tachycardia, advanced or high-degree AV block, bundle branch block.** This ECG strip from the same patient in Figure 48. There is a regular sinus P wave at a rate of about 107 bpm. The QRS is wide with an irregular ventricular rhythm. You need a caliper to "march-out" the P waves in this case. Some of the P waves are "partly hidden from view" or some of the P waves are merging with the descending component of the T waves. The partially hidden P waves are marked with arrows. The P wave distortion can also be seen on V1 (arrows). In this case, mostly 2 P waves are not conducted and only one P wave is conducted or followed by a QRS. The pattern is that of 2:1 and 3:1. *Most likely you will not see these kinds of strips in basic ECG test.* If you see this, others would label it as second degree AV block type II (Mobitz II).

Third Degree AV Block

Third degree AV block is also called complete heart block (CHB). The supraventricular impulse is totally blocked from reaching the ventricles. The atria and ventricles beats independently.

ECG Recognition:

- In sinus rhythm with complete AV block, the PP and RR intervals are regular but the P wave has no relationship with the R wave.
- The PR interval varies because there is really no P and QRS relationship.
- The ventricular rate is usually 40-60 bpm and narrow when it is driven by a junctional pacemaker (AV node).
- The QRS is wide and less the 40 bpm when an infra-Hisian pacemaker takes over.

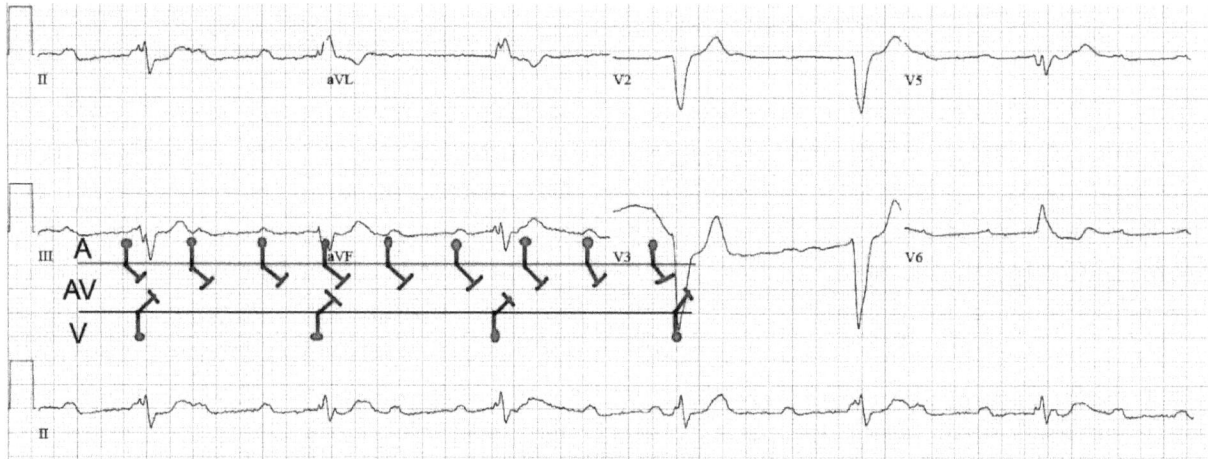

Figure 56 - **Sinus tachycardia, complete heart block with idioventricular escape rhythm.** There is a regular sinus P wave at a rate of about 107 bpm. There is regular wide QRS rhythm of about 38 bpm. The PRI varies. Hence, the P wave has no relationship to the QRS. A ladder diagram or laddergram is shown on the left to illustrate sinus impulse from the A or atrial tier/level is blocked in AV or atrioventricular junction tier/level. The laddergram also shows the ventricles are depolarized from the ventricular or V tier (infra-Hisian pacemaker). The reason for a wide QRS in ventricular escape rhythm is because muscle to muscle conduction is slow.

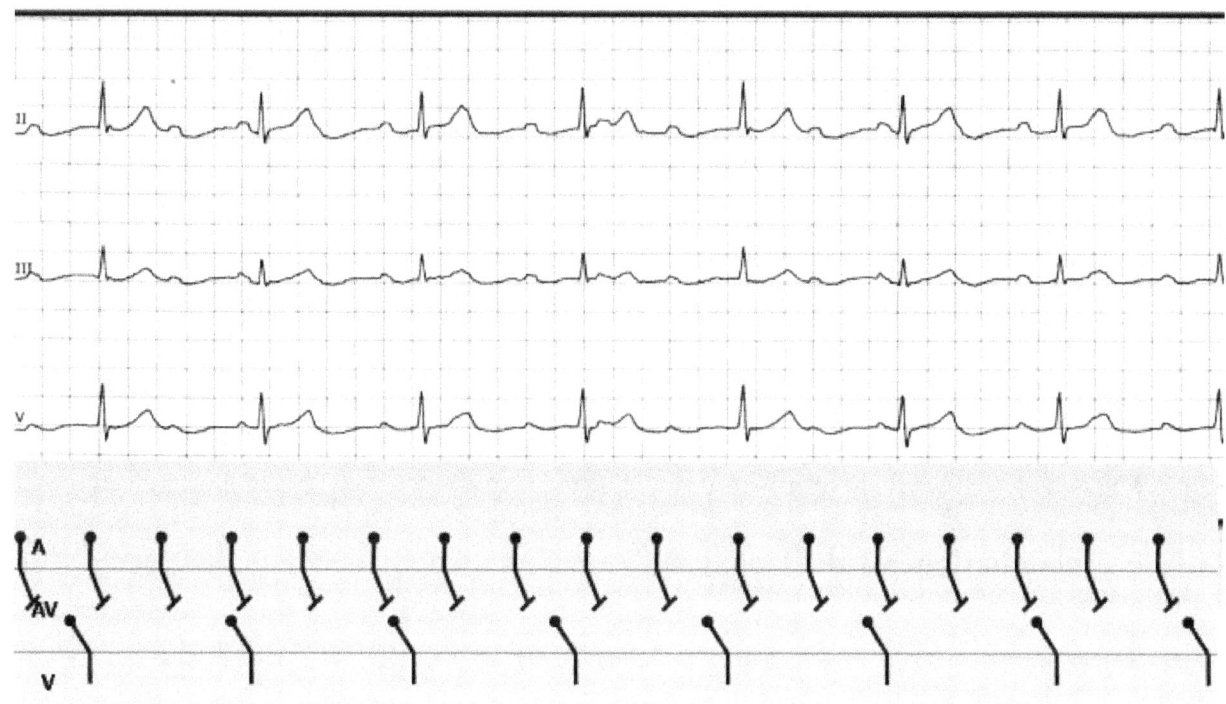

Figure 57 - **Sinus tachycardia, complete heart block with junctional escape rhythm.** There is a regular sinus P wave at a rate of about 125 bpm and regular narrow QRS complex rhythm of about 55 bpm. There is no relationship between the P and QRS which showed variable PRI. The reason for a narrow QRS in junctional escape rhythm is because of faster conduction via the normal conduction pathway (AV junction to the His-purkinje system).

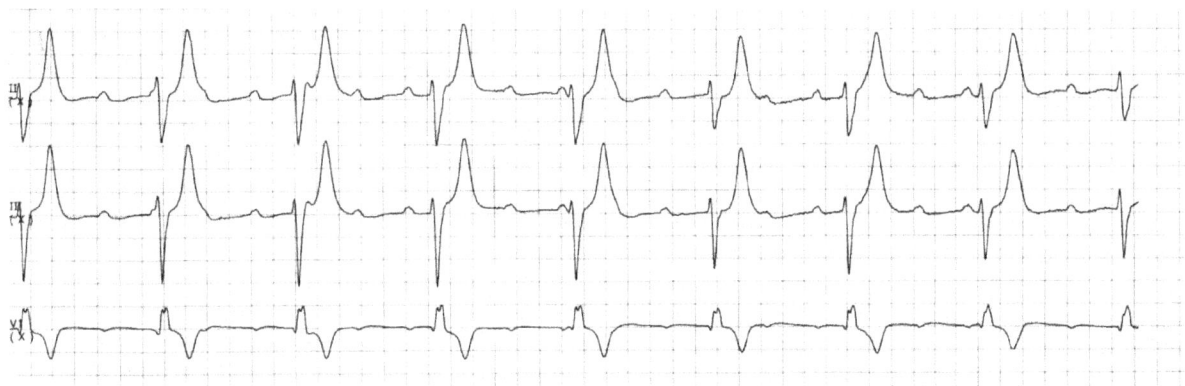

Figure 58 - **Sinus tachycardia, complete heart block, accelerated idioventricular escape rhythm (AIVR).** There is a regular sinus P wave at a rate of about 125 bpm and a regular wide QRS complex rhythm at a rate of about 46 bpm. There is no relationship between the P and QRS.

Paroxysmal AV block (ventricular standstill)

ECG Recognition:

- It is characterized by an abrupt and persistent AV block (multiple P waves with no QRS) in the presence of otherwise normal AV conduction.
- It may be initiated by a conducted or blocked PAC or PVC, acceleration or slowing of sinus rhythm.
- Once the block is initiated, the block will persist until terminated by an escape, usually ventricular, with a predictable relationship of the escape to the following P wave.

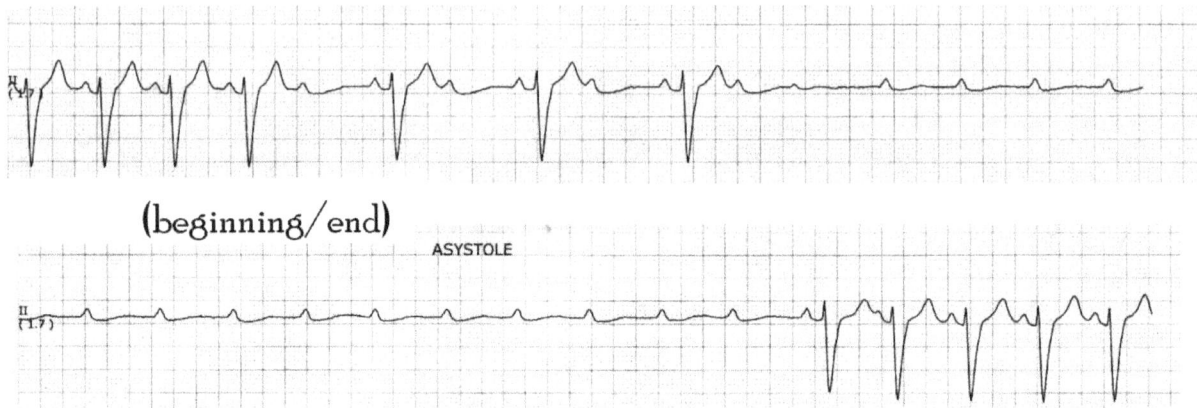

Figure 59 - Continuous lead II strip of **Paroxysmal AV block or ventricular standstill**

Atrial Flutter

Atrial flutter (AFL) is an arrhythmia that can be likened to a dog chasing its tail creating a circus movement (reentrant arrhythmia). The impulse travels from the interatrial septum to the right atrial free wall. The impulse can travel clockwise or counter-clockwise.

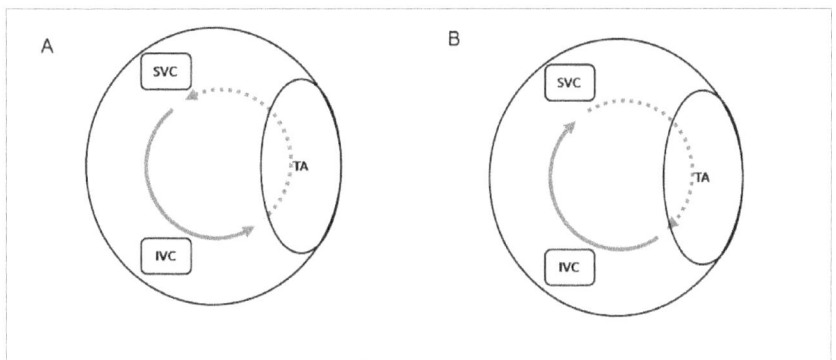

Figure 60 - Figures A and B shows the simplified counter-clockwise and clockwise movement of atrial flutter in the right atrium. SVC - superior vena cava, IVC - inferior vena cava, TA - atrial septum

ECG Recognition:

- Typical AFL waves are best seen in II, III and aVF (inferior leads) which have a regular rhythm, and constant morphology.
- **There is a downsloping segment followed by a sharper negative deflection, and then a sharp positive deflection, with a positive overshoot leading to the next downsloping plateau (sawtooth).**
- Typical clockwise is the inversion of the appearance in counter-clockwise AF with broad positive deflections in the inferior leads and a wide negative deflection in V1.
- Typical AFL rate is usually 240-340 bpm but can be slower in patients on antiarrhythmics, atrial myopathy or patients who had incomplete ablation.
- Most commonly there is 2:1 AV conduction but variable conduction (4:1 or 6:1) can be seen.
- The QRs morphology will look the same during sinus rhythm unless there is aberrancy.

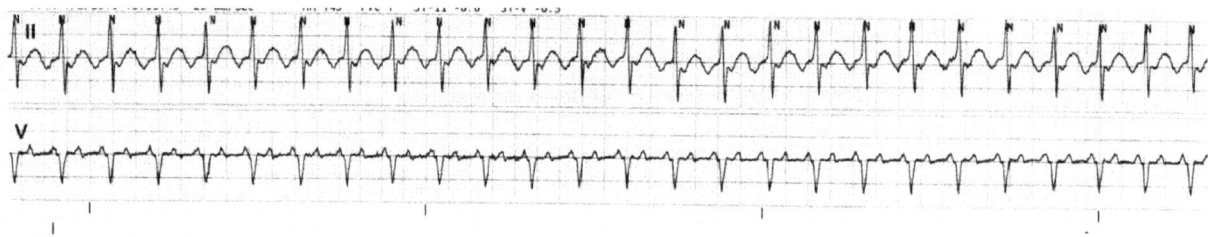

Figure 61 - Counter-clockwise **atrial flutter** with 2:1 AV conduction. Sawtooth pattern seen in lead II and atrial rate best at 300 bpm and atrial activity best seen in V1.

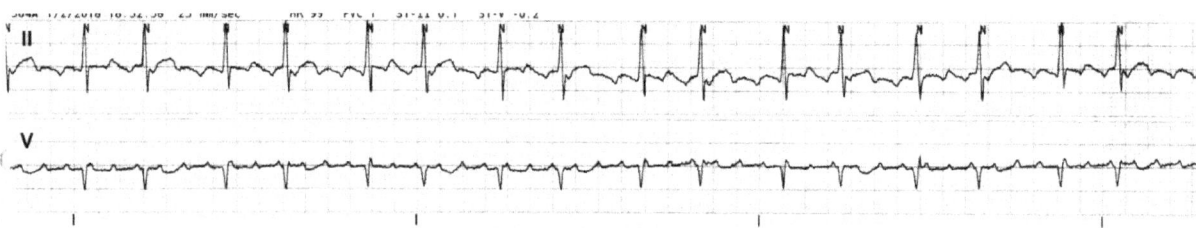

Figure 62 - **Atrial flutter with variable AV conduction.** Sawtooth pattern seen on lead II and atrial flutter rate best computed using PP interval in V1 with 1 big square (~300 bpm).

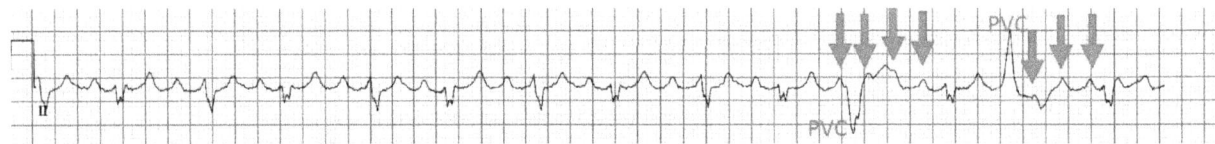

Figure 63 - Clockwise **atrial flutter** unmasked by a properly-timed PVC. The 2 multifocal PVC exposed the hidden P waves (arrows).

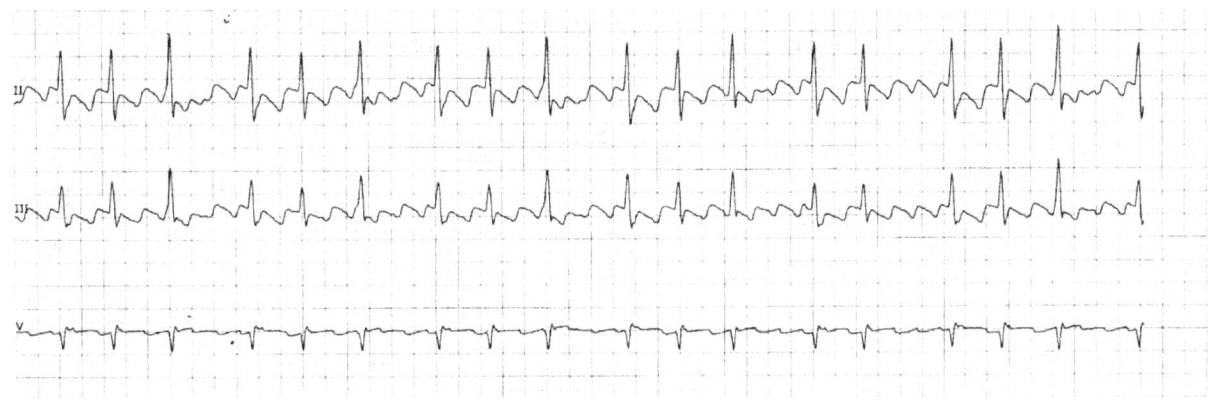

Figure 64 - **Atrial flutter with variable AV conduction.** This is an irregular narrow QRS complex rhythm with flutter waves in II and III. The flutter rate is about 300 bpm.

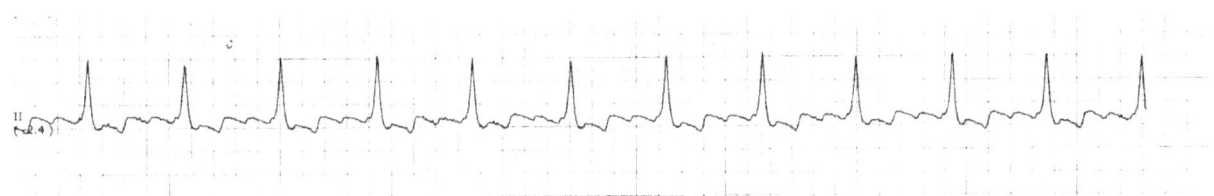

Figure 65 - **Atrial flutter with 4:1 AV conduction.** This is a regular wide QRS complex rhythm at a ventricular rate of about 70 bpm with flutter waves. There are 4 flutter waves for every 1 QRS (4:1 AV conduction).

Atrial Tachycardia

Most basic ECG test will not have atrial tachycardia but this is a common paroxysmal atrial arrhythmia encountered. It is inserted after atrial flutter because as mentioned before the rate of atrial flutter (around 250-350 bpm) can become slower in patients taking antiarrhytmics, patients with atrial myopathy and patients who had incomplete ablation. So, it becomes difficult to differentiate slow atrial flutter from atrial tachycardia.

ECG Recognition:

- The heart rate may be as low as 100 to as high as 240 bpm and rhythm is regular.
- The contour of the P wave depends on the site of origin. The P wave is different during sinus rhythm but may look like the appearance during sinus rhythm if the origin is near the SA node. It may also be low amplitude or negative in II, III and aVF.
- The PRI may be normal or prolonged.
- The AV conduction ratio may be 1:1 at rates about 240 bpm.
- At rapid rates, there may be an AV block (atrial tachycardia with a block) because the impulse will encounter the AV node in the refractory period.
- The AV block can be 2:1 or the ratio may be higher.
- A Wenckebach block is common.

*It is easier to identify atrial tachycardia in monitored patients because you can catch the beginning, middle and end/termination of the arrhythmia. The heart rate histogram is also a valuable tool to determine if you are dealing with sinus tachycardia or atrial tachycardia. Sinus tachycardia will have a gradual increase and decrease in heart rate but it will be a sudden increase and decrease for atrial tachycardia.

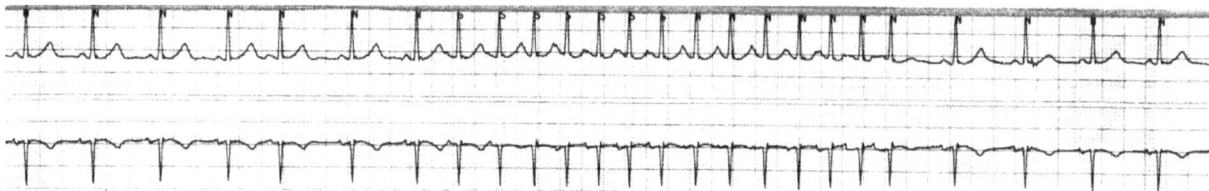

Figure 66 - **Paroxysmal atrial tachycardia.** There is sudden onset and termination of narrow QRS complex tachycardia with distinct P waves best seen in V1.

Atrial Fibrillation

Atrial fibrillation (AF) is a supraventricular arrhythmia.

ECG Recognition:

Atrial Activity
- It is seen as oscillations of low amplitude (f waves) at a rate of about 300-600 bpm.
- These waves have variable amplitude, shape and timing.
- Sometimes, f waves can mimic atrial flutter in V1. There is absence of uniform and regular atrial activity in other leads in AF compared to AFL.
- In some, the f waves are so small. The diagnosis of atrial fibrillation on these patients will be based on the irregularly irregular ventricular activity.

Ventricular activity
- Irregularly irregular ventricular rhythm.
- About 100-160 bpm in the absence of drugs affecting the AV node.
- Typically called AF with rapid ventricular response (AF with RVR) if the ventricular rate is > 100 bpm and AF with slow ventricular response if ventricular rate is < 60 bpm.
- Can be more than 250 bpm in the presence accessory pathway in cases of Wolff-Parkinson-White (WPW) syndrome
- Can look regular when the rate is more than 170 bpm.
- Can be regular in cases of paced beats and complete heart block with regular escape beats.
- QRS can be narrow or wide if there is an existing bundle branch block or aberrancy.

In basic ECG test, the typical strip will show fibrillatory waves which could be fine or coarse and an irregularly irregular ventricular rhythm.

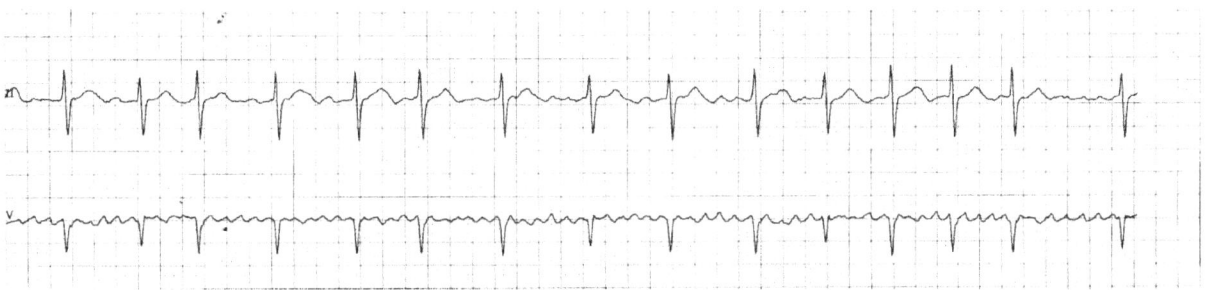

Figure 67 - **Atrial fibrillation.** Course fibrillatory waves seen in V1.

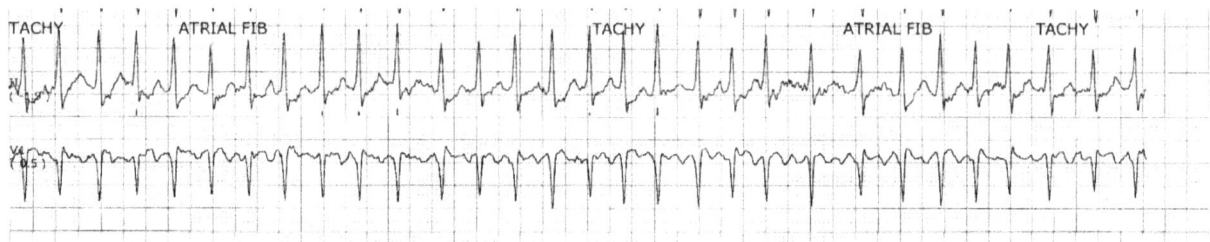

Figure 68 - **Atrial fibrillation with rapid ventricular response.** This is an irregularly irregular narrow QRS complex tachycardia at a rate of about 180 bpm. Coarse fibrillatory waves can be seen in V1.

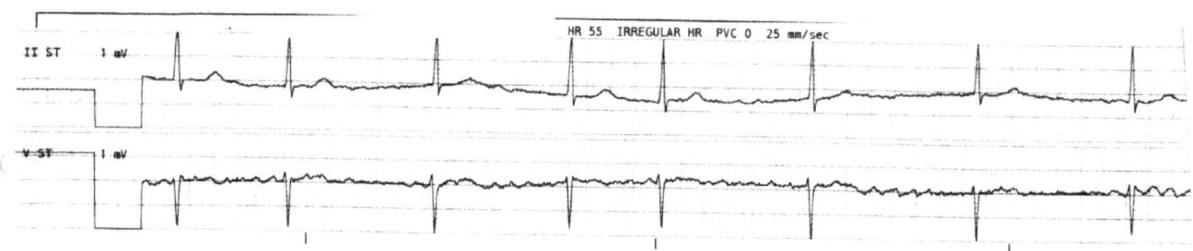

Figure 69 - **Atrial fibrillation with slow ventricular response.** Fine fibrillatory waves with ventricular rate of about 50 bpm (rate computed using the 6-second method).

Supraventricular Tachycardia

In basic ECG test, the acceptable answer for a regular narrow QRS complex tachycardia with no visible P waves is supraventricular tachycardia (SVT).

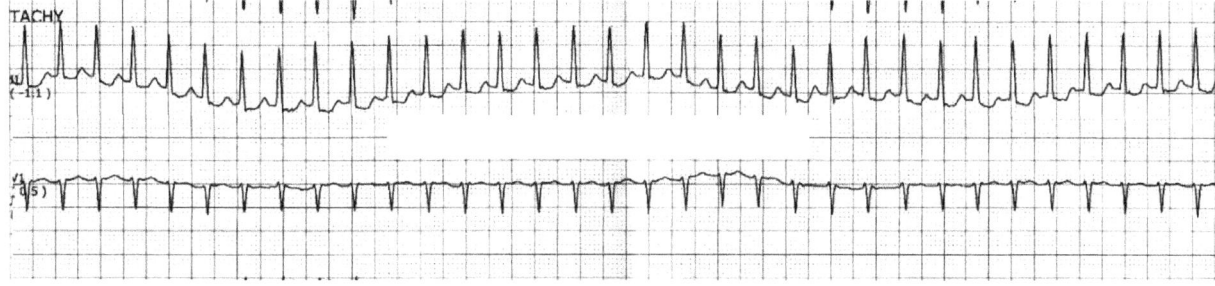

Figure 70 - **Supraventricular tachycardia**. This is a regular narrow QRS complex tachycardia with no visible P waves.

But what is a SVT?

Supraventricular tachycardia (SVT) is the term often given for a narrow complex tachycardia with no identifiable P waves. However, SVT is a general term for a group of arrhythmia with the impulse originating above (supra - Latin for above) the ventricles which could either be the sinus node, atria, AV node or the bundle of His.

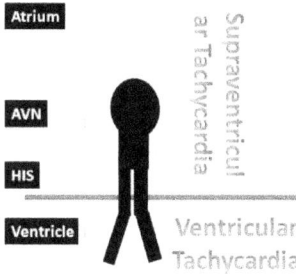

Figure 71 - Diagram classifying tachycardia into supraventricular tachycardia and ventricular tachycardia.

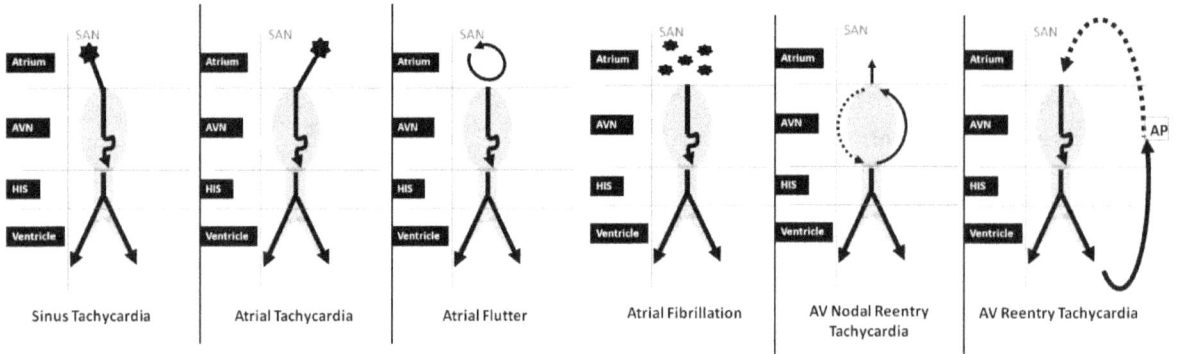

Figure 72 - Simplified diagram of SVT. This is a nice to know for basic ECG test.

All of the above arrhythmia will look like a SVT on a typical ECG test. It will be beyond this guide to discuss all the arrhythmia.

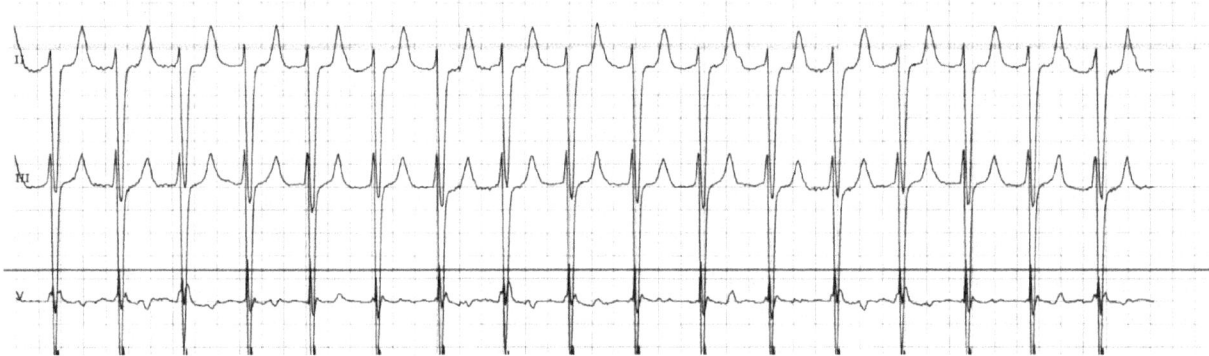

Figure 73 - **Supraventricular tachycardia.** A 3 lead ECG strip of regular wide QRS complex tachycardia. It is difficult to spot the P waves. However, by closer inspection, P waves are seen to merge with the T waves which are best seen in lead II as shown below.

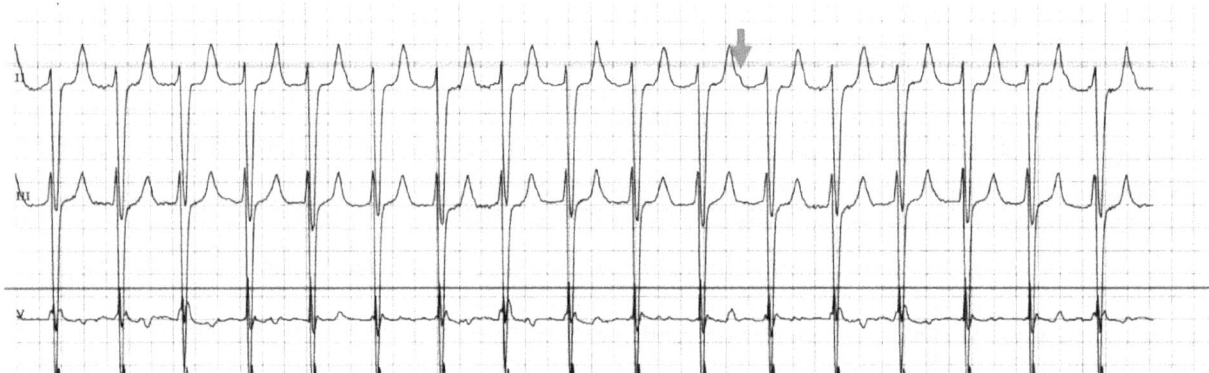

Figure 74 - **Supraventricular tachycardia** which is actually **atrial tachycardia.** It is difficult to tell from this strip but catching the initiation will make the diagnosis easy (Figure 75). Most, if not all, basic ECG test will not show this ECG strip.

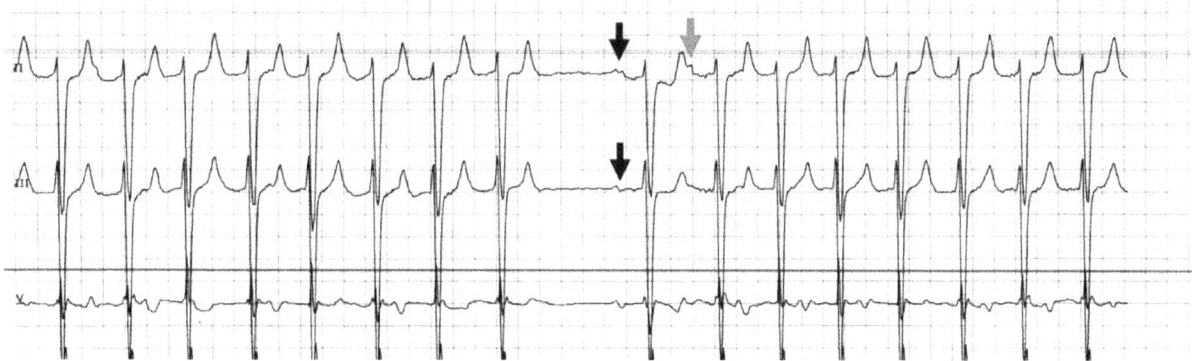

Figure 75 - The initiation or beginning ECG strip of atrial tachycardia. Sinus P wave is marked with arrows in lead II and III. A distinct P wave marked with an arrow after the sinus P wave is the start of the atrial tachycardia. From there, the P wave is difficult to see.

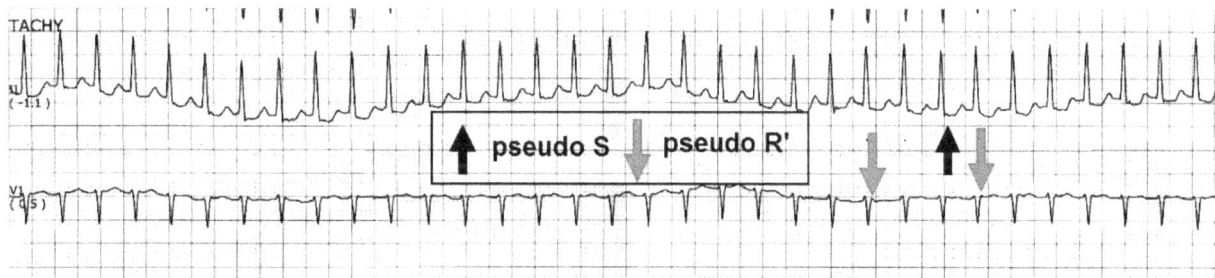

Figure 76 - **Supraventricular tachycardia (SVT)** - AV nodal reentry tachycardia. This the same ECG strip in Figure 70. The pseudo R and pseudo S are challenging for beginners but can be appreciated by skilled ECG readers. If you go back to the AV nodal reentry diagram in Figure 72, the pseudo-S and pseudo R are the retrograde depolarization of the atrium as the impulse go up. If ever an ECG like this appear in basic ECG test, supraventricular tachycardia or SVT is an acceptable answer. arrow pointing up- pseudo S, arrow pointing down - pseudo R.

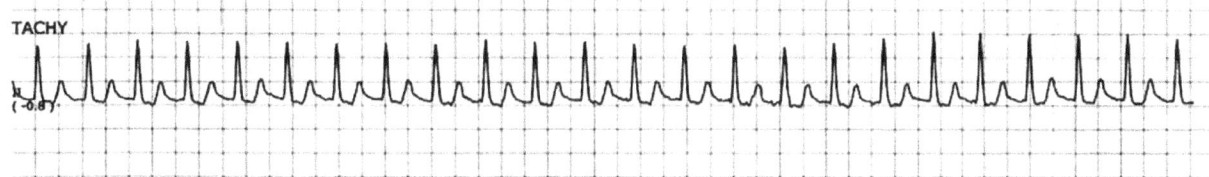

Figure 77 - **Supraventricular tachycardia (SVT)**. This is actually sinus tachycardia with the P waves merged with the T waves. In this ECG strip, it is difficult to tell what kind of SVT. Thus, for testing purposes, once you see this, the answer is SVT.

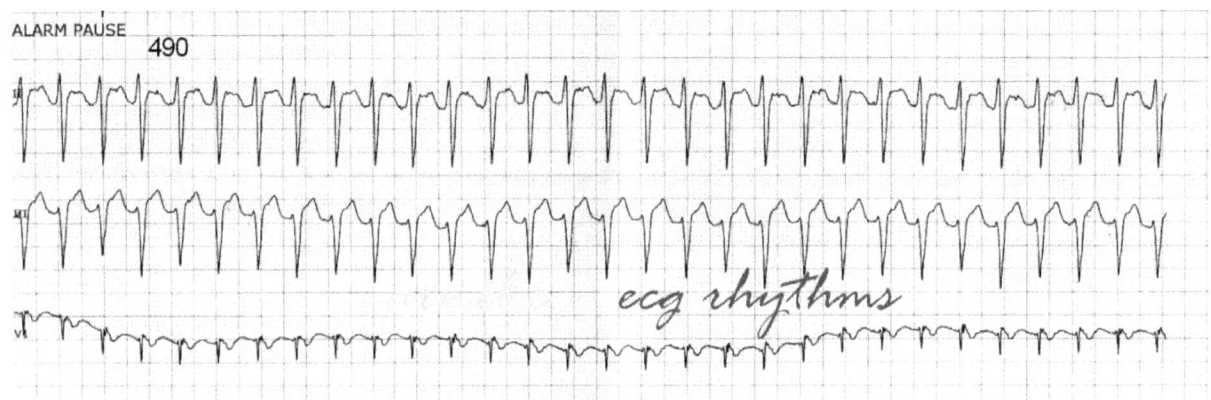

Figure 78 - **Supraventricular tachycardia (SVT).** This is a 3-lead ECG strip of a regular narrow QRS complex tachycardia. P waves are difficult to see.

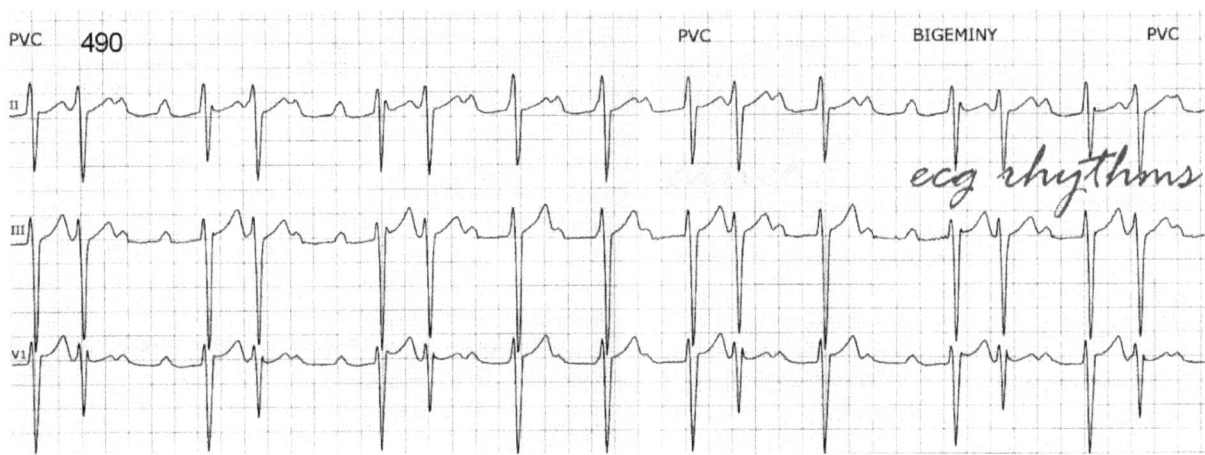

Figure 79 - This is the 3-lead ECG strip of the case above at a slower ventricular rate. The SVT in Figure 78 turned-out to be **atrial tachycardia vs. atrial flutter** (slow). It is difficult to tell by certainty atrial flutter (slow) from atrial tachycardia on the surface ECG alone. An electrophysiology study can determine which is which. You will not see this kind of ECG strip in basic ECG test. So, don't worry. This is just to highlight that an SVT can be any tachycardia with the impulse originating above the ventricles.

Ventricular Rhythms

Ventricular rhythm or arrhythmia is recognized on the surface ECG as wide QRS (>0.12 sec) rhythms with direction of the QRS and T wave opposite each other. So, when the QRS is predominantly pointing upward (positive) then the T wave is pointing downward (negative). The P wave has no relationship with the wide QRS (if present) and vice-versa.

It is sometimes difficult to differentiate ventricular arrhythmia from aberrancy or intermittent abnormal widening of the QRS. In most basic ECG test, most wide QRS rhythms with no P waves are ventricular arrhythmia.

Premature Ventricular Complexes (PVC)

Premature ventricular complex (PVC) are also known by several names: premature ventricular beat, ventricular ectopic beats, ventricular ectopy, ventricular extrasystole and ventricular premature depolarization. However, the most popular name or commonly known name is PVC od premature ventricular complex.

ECG Recognition:

- This wide QRS beats comes in early or premature in relation to the intrinsic rhythm.
- The QRS and T wave are pointing opposite each other.
- There is *usually* a full compensatory pause after the PVC.
- An inverted or retrograde P wave may or may not be seen.
- PVC can occur in a pattern just like premature atrial complex as mentioned before (bigeminy, trigeminy and so on).
- If the shapes of the PVC's are the same then it is called monomophic PVC but if the shapes are different then it is called polymorphic PVC's.
- If a PVC appear in pairs then is it called couplet. Three PVC's in succession is called triplet or already called ventricular tachycardia (non-sustained).

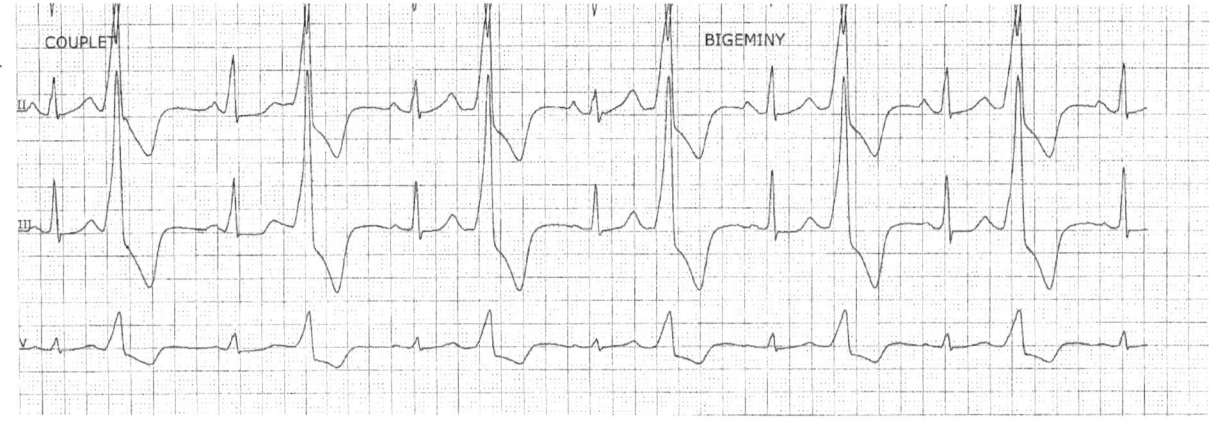

Figure 80 - **Premature ventricular complex in bigeminy.** Every other normal beat is followed by a wide QRS complex.

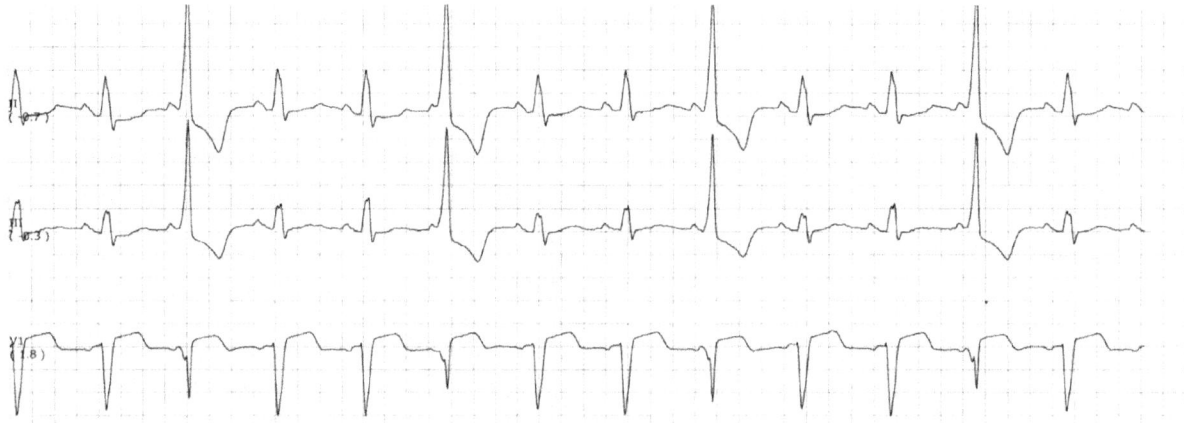

Figure 81 - **PVC in trigeminy.** Every 2 sinus beats with wide QRS complexes or bundle branch block morphology is followed with a wider QRS complex with no relationship to the P wave.

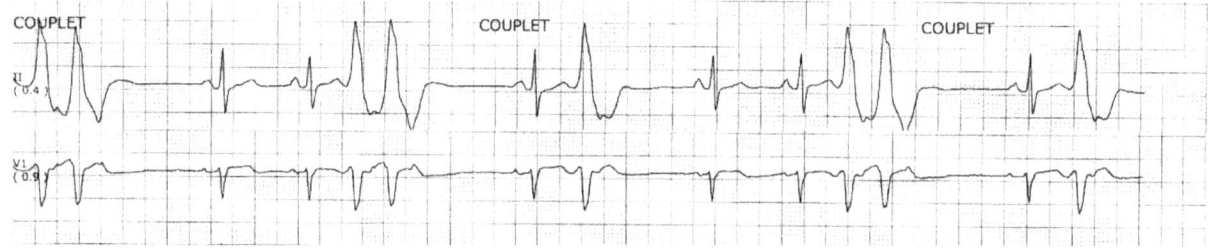

Figure 82 - **PVC's in couplet.** Two wide QRS beats that appear in succession is called couplet. If the PVC's appear in 3, then it is called triplet or ventricular tachycardia.

Idioventricular Rhythm and accelerated idioventricular rhythm

If the impulse from normal sinus pacemaker or the junctional pacemaker fails to reach the ventricles, the next pacemaker (ventricles) kicks-in or the ventricle "escapes" from the typical sinoatrial node control.

ECG Recognition:

- These are regular wide QRS complexes with rates around 30-40 bpm.
- The rate may be as slow as 20 or as high as 50 bpm.
- If the rate is between 60-100 bpm, it is called accelerated idioventricular rhythm

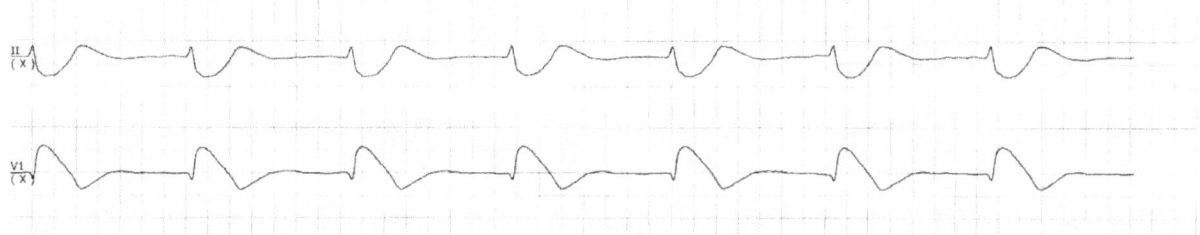

Figure 83 - **Idioventricular rhythm.** This is a regular very wide QRS rhythm at a rate of about 40 bpm.

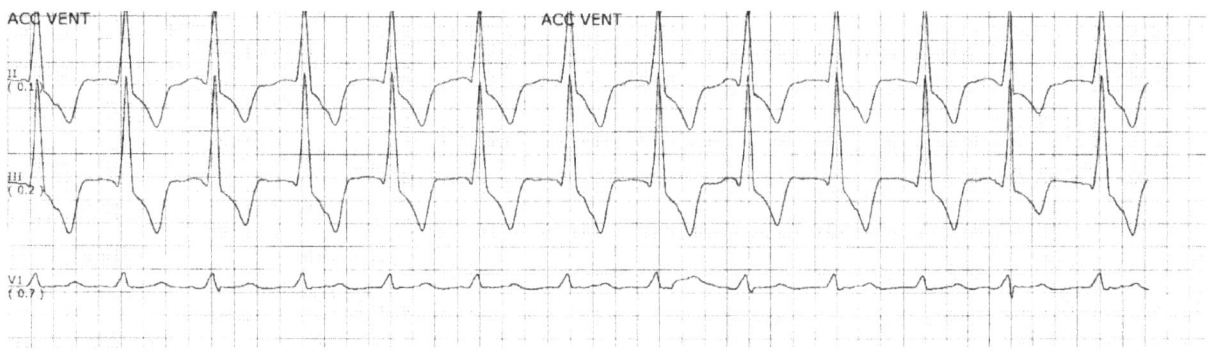

Figure 84 - **Accelerated idioventricular rhythm.** This is a regular wide QRS rhythm at a rate of about 75 bpm.

Ventricular Tachycardia (VT)

If there is a rapid succession of 3 or more PVC's then it is called ventricular tachycardia.

If the tachycardia is more than 30 seconds, it is called sustained VT and non-sustained VT if less than 30 seconds.

In basic ECG test, you are only shown a 6 second or 10 second strip. So, it is hard to tell if is sustained. Most of the time the whole strip will be filled with wide QRS complexes and it will be labeled ventricular tachycardia.

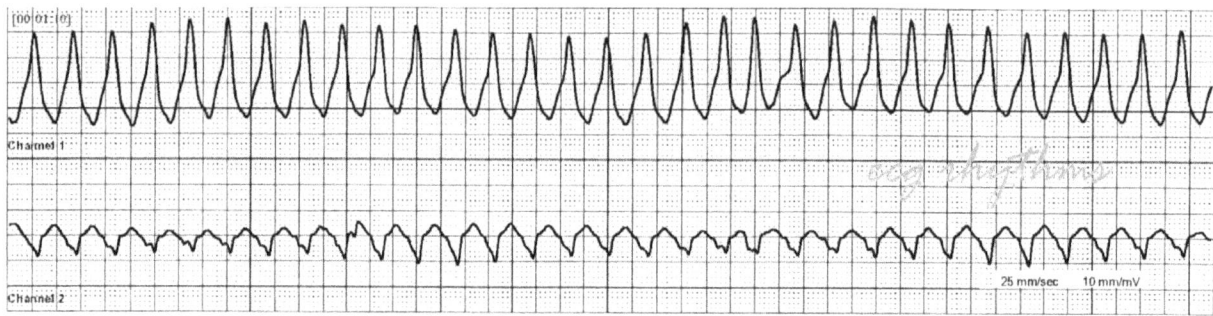

Figure 85 - **Ventricular tachycardia**. This is a regular monomorphic (same-shape) wide complex rhythm at a rate of about 214 bpm.

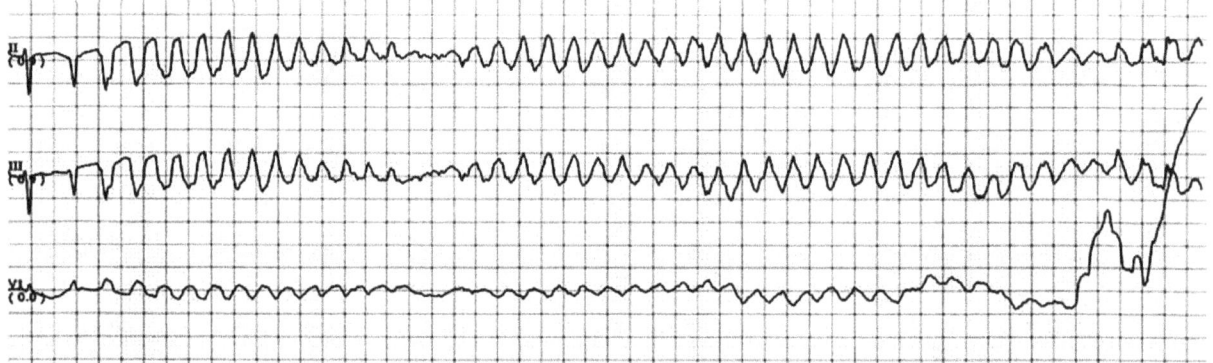

Figure 86 - **Ventricular tachycardia**. This is a regular polymorphic (different shape QRS) wide complex rhythm at a rate of about 300 bpm. This is from a patient with ischemic cardiomyopathy with an ejection fraction of 25%.

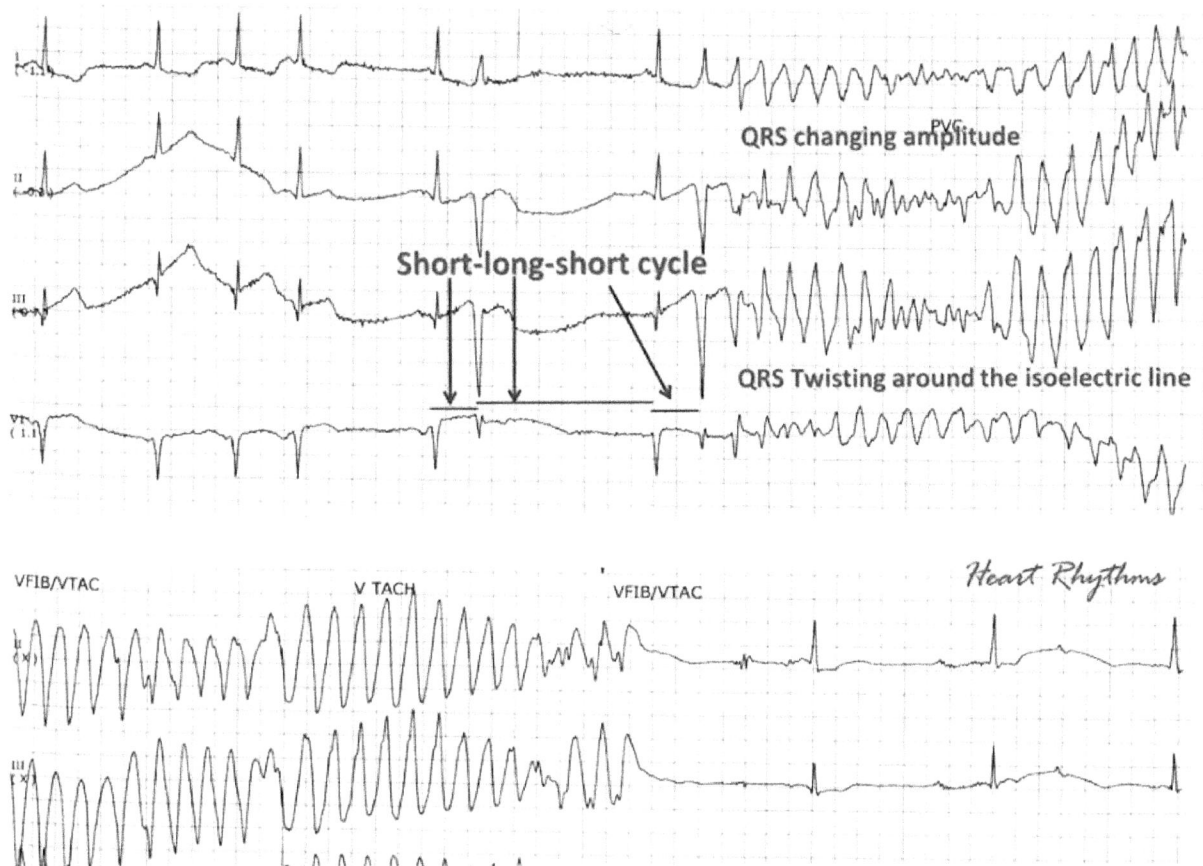

Figure 87 - The upper ECG strip is the typical initiation of **Torsades de Pointes**. This highlights the short R to R then long RR and short RR cycle or the short-long-short RR cycle. The typical twisting of the QRS complex is then seen with the abrupt termination in the lower strip. If you see an ECG strip in a basic ECG test that "twist" or has a changing polarity of the QRS, then the *expected answer is Torsades de Pointes or TdP*. However, TdP should only be used if it is known that there is an existing prolonged QTc. Otherwise, if you cannot determine of the strip that there is a prolonged QTc, then it is called polymoprhic VT.

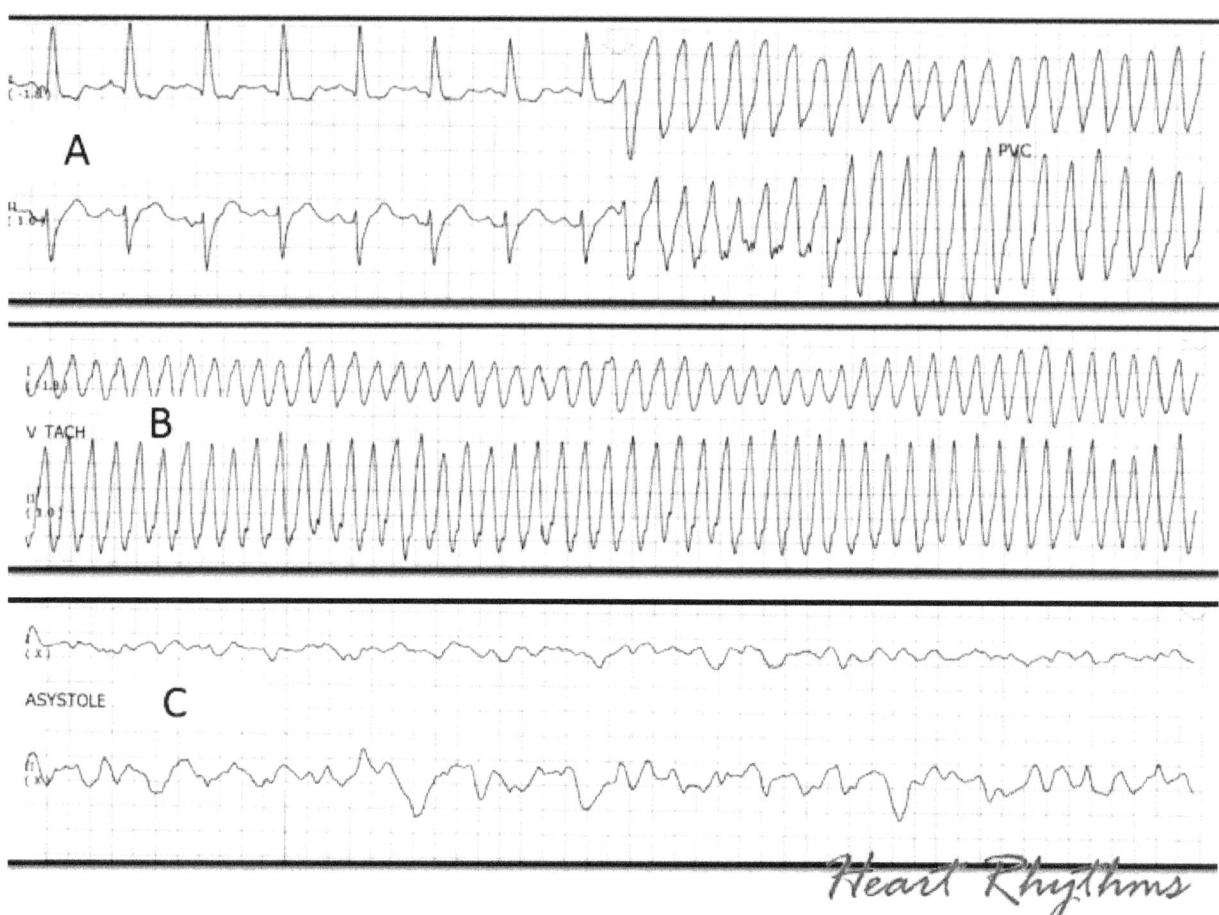

Figure 88 - **Monomorphic VT, ventricular flutter, ventricular fibrillation.** A - Ventricular tachycardia - Onset of a fast monomorphic VT with a rate of about 250 bpm. B - Ventricular flutter- Lead II looked like sinusoidal pattern with a rate of about 300 bpm. C Ventricular fibrillation- undulations of varying contour and amplitude noted with absence of organized QRST waves. Distinction between fast ventricular tachycardia and ventricular flutter is difficult and is usually of academic interest. These are fatal arrhythmias and interventions must be done promptly.

Paced Rhythms

Pacemakers are device that serve as a back-up mechanism if all things fail. You will then see the obvious pacemaker spikes/artifact on the ECG strip. If after an R wave, the next R wave is not seen then the pacemaker delivers a stimulus. Pacemaker stimulus is sometimes called pacer artifact or spike.

ECG test on paced rhythms will most likely be only atrial and ventricular pacing strips, failure to pace, failure to capture and undersensing.

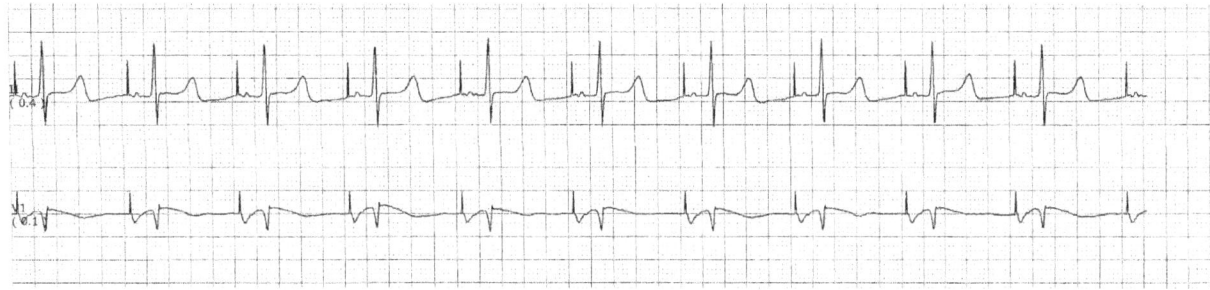

Figure 89- **Atrial paced or A-paced.** Pacer spikes noted before the P waves. The QRS is narrow because it is intrinsic.

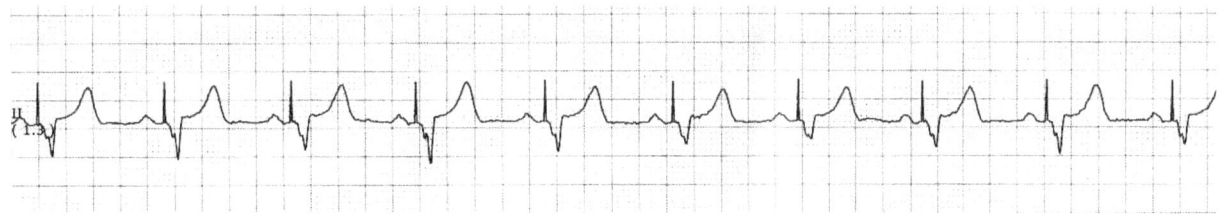

Figure 90 - **Ventricular pacing or V-pacing.** There is an intrinsic sinus P wave that is sensed by the machine. A pacemaker artifact is noted before the wide QRS indicating the pacemaker delivered the impulse depolarizing the ventricles.

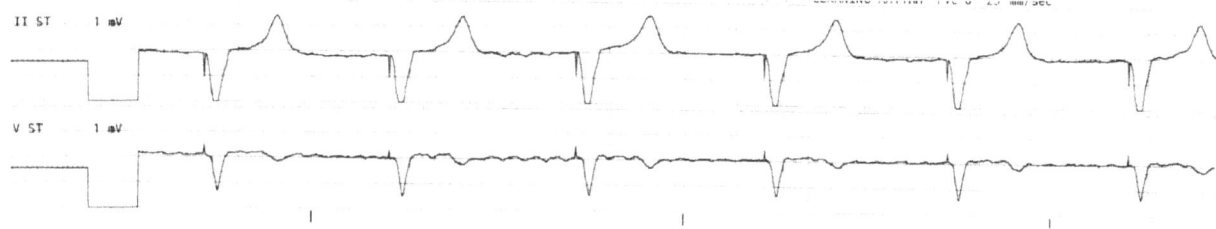

Figure 91 - **Ventricular pacing at 40 bpm, atrial fibrillation.** Pacemakers can sometimes be set at a lower limit about 40 bpm. Also, in this case, fibrillatory waves are seen which indicate that the intrinsic rhythm atrial fibrillation.

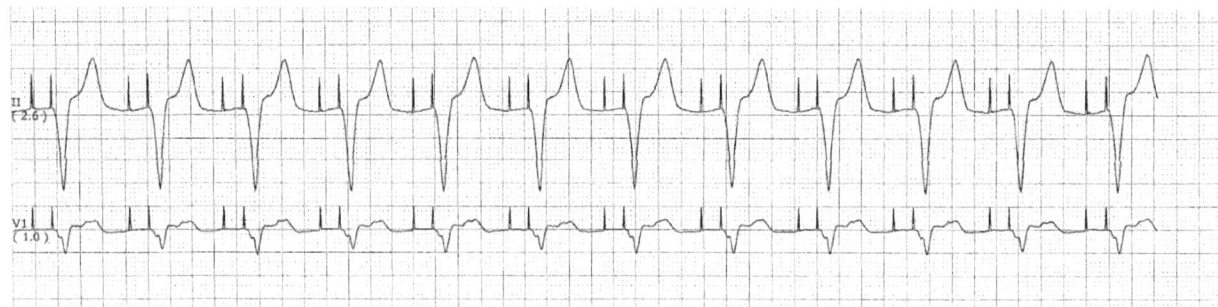

Figure 92 - **AV pacing**. Two pacemaker spikes are seen indicating dual chamber pacing (atrium and ventricle).

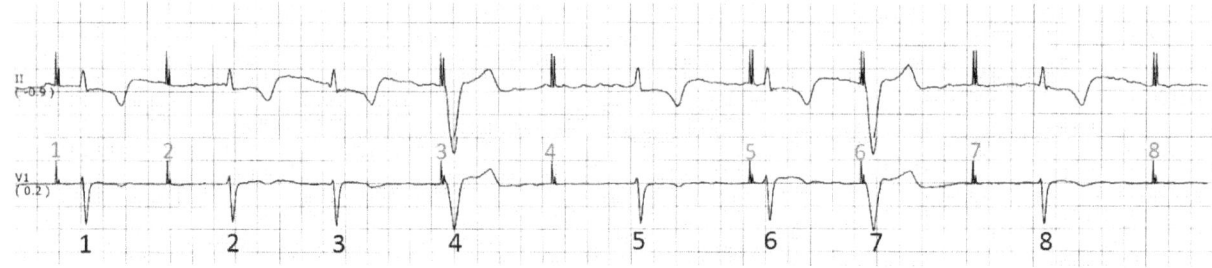

Figure 93 - **Atrial fibrillation with slow ventricular response in a patient with VVI pacemaker, Intermittent failure to capture or loss of capture and intermittent undersensing**. Pacemaker artifacts are set at a rate of about 60 bpm (1500/25 small squares or 1,000 ms cycle in pacemaker terms). This is obviously seen in pacemaker spike #3 creating wide QRS #4. Pacemaker spikes # 1,2,4,5,7 and 8 were not followed by a wide QRS. So, those pacer artifacts failed to capture the ventricle. Pacemaker artifacts # 3 and 6 (capture) were followed by a wide QRS. So, the pacemaker was intermittently failing to capture. The second problem seen is intermittent undersensing. Pacemaker artifacts #3,4,5,7 and 8 were pacer impulse fired 1,000 ms (5 small squares) after a QRS. Thus, QRS # 3,4,5,7 and 8 were sensed by the pacemaker. However, pacer artifact #2 and 6 can be noted to fired earlier than 1,000 ms (5 small boxes). Thus, the pacemaker was intermittently undersensing those QRS (# 1 and 6) complexes. Fibrillatory waves can be noted. The intrinsic rhythm is atrial fibrillation with a narrow QRS complex.

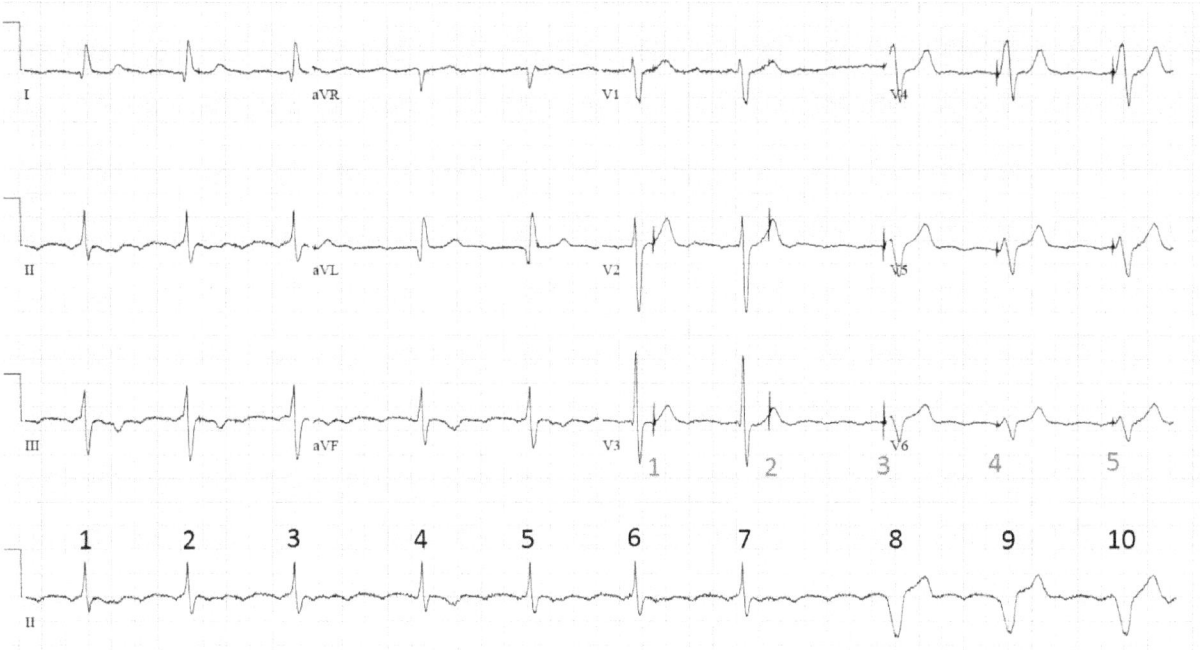

Figure 94 - **Atrial flutter in patient with VVI pacemaker, failure to sense and functional non-capture.** You will not see 12-lead ECG in a basic ECG test and all pacer spikes are visible and not unlike in this ECG strip. So, do not worry. This case is presented to highlight failure to sense and functional non-capture. The intrinsic rhythm is atrial flutter with inverted P wave best seen in lead II. Pacer spikes (labeled with red numbers) are best seen in V1 to V6 but not in lead II. This is because this due to bipolar pacing. Bipolar pacing will generate a tiny or small pacer spike compared to unipolar pacing. As mentioned, do not worry because most ECG test will show those pacer spikes in lead II. You will see tiny pacer spikes in the real world. Since we cannot definitely see if there are pacer spikes between QRS #1-6, we will focus on pacer spike # 1 and 2. QRS # 6 and 7 are not sense (failure to sense). Pacer spike # 1 and 2 is not a "real" non-capture but a "functional" non-capture. This is because the pacer spike was delivered during the physiologic refractory period of the ventricle. There is no way for the ventricle to be depolarized during this period. Thus, the main problem here is failure to sense.

Review

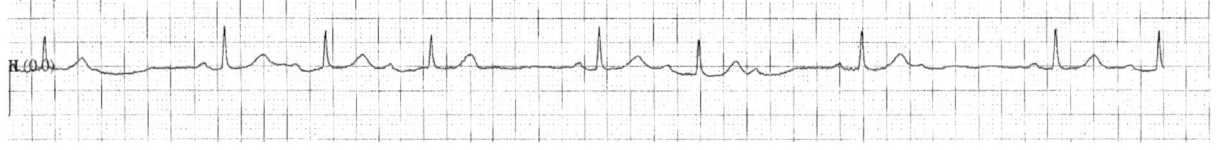

1. _____

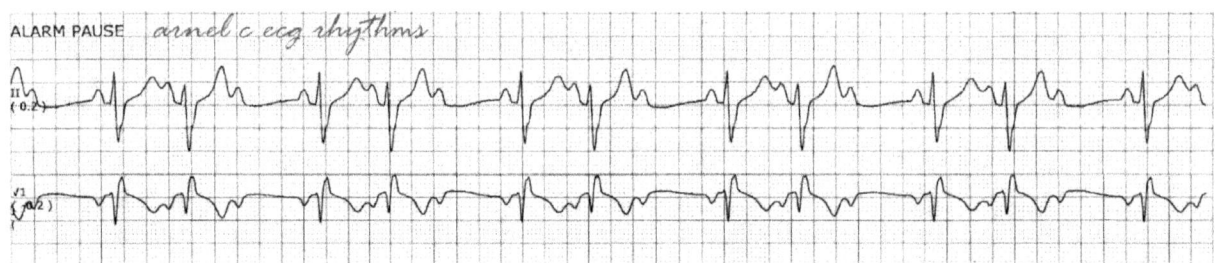

2. _____

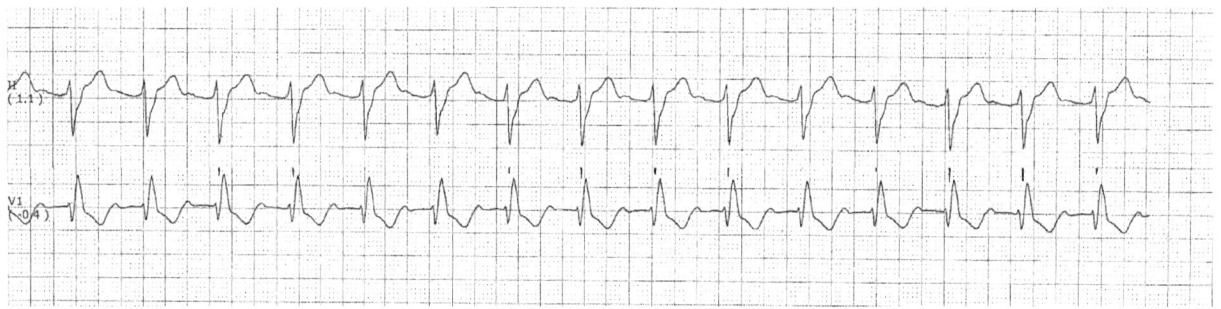

3. _____

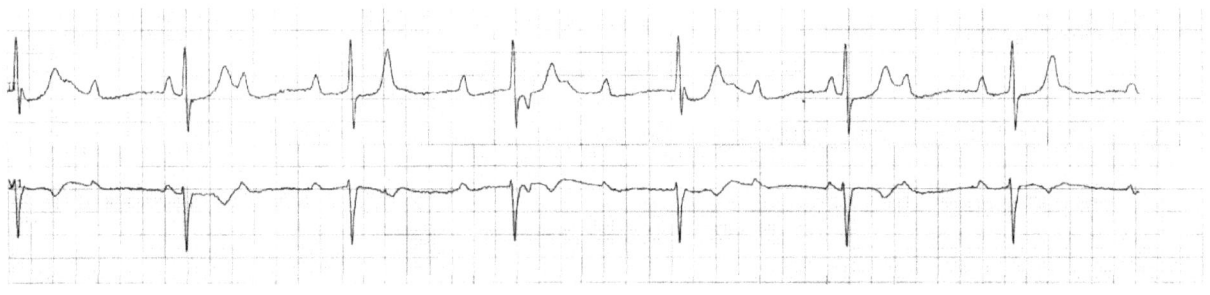

4. _____

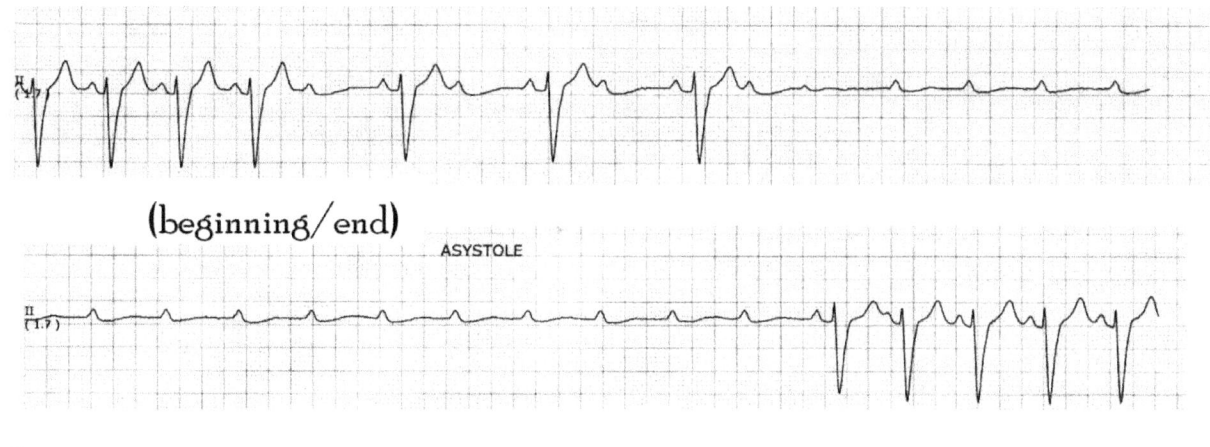

(beginning/end)

ASYSTOLE

5. _____

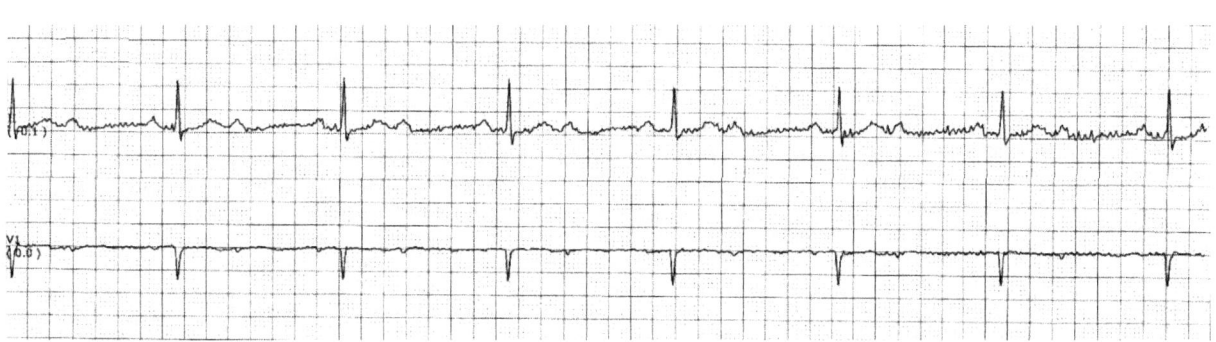

6. _____

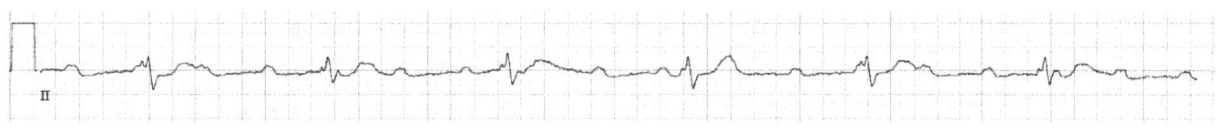

7. _____

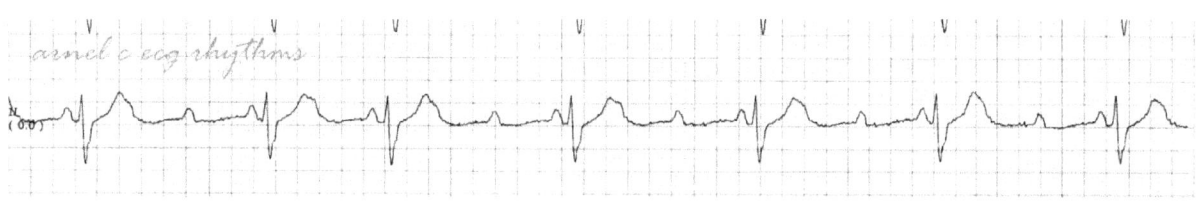

8. _____

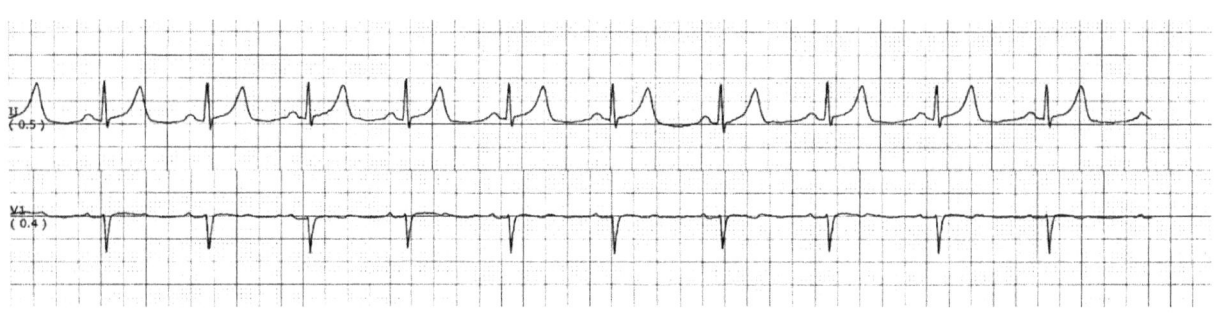

9. _____

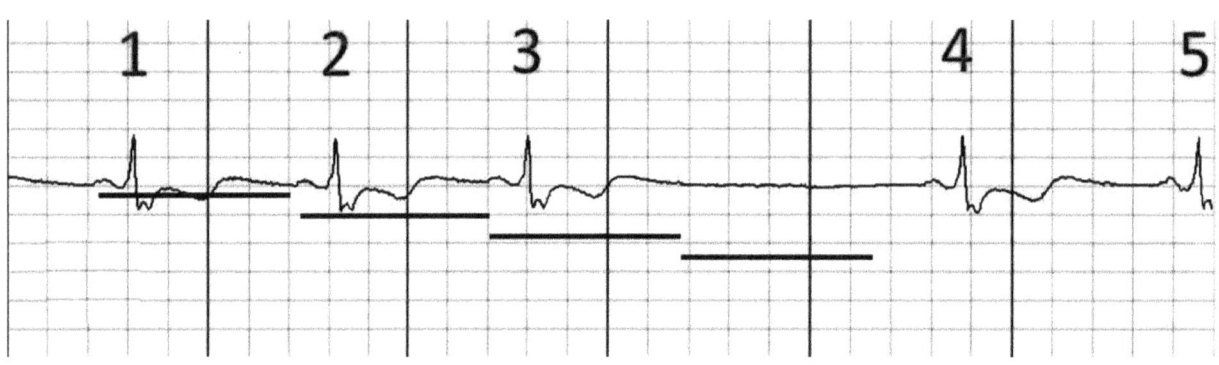

10. _____

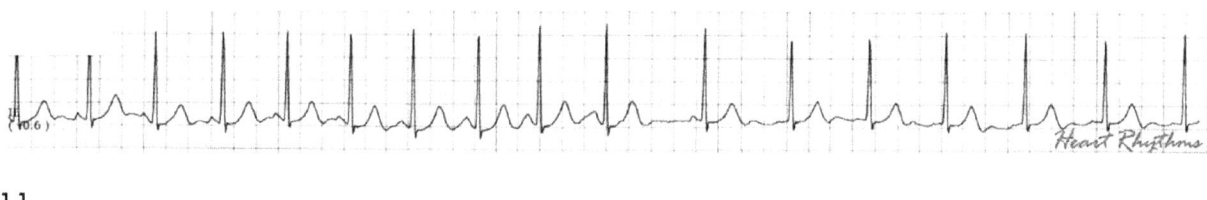

11. _____

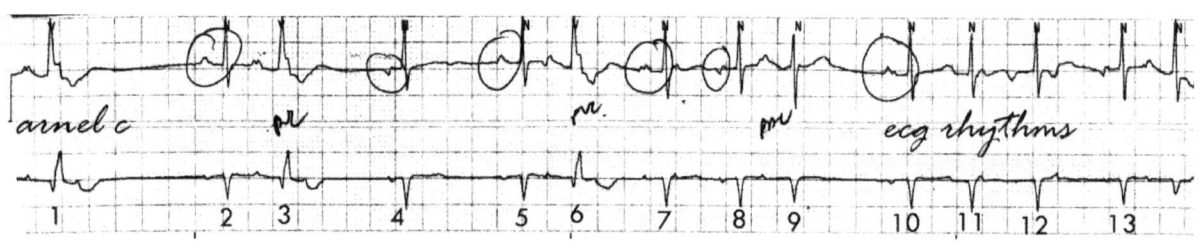

12. _____

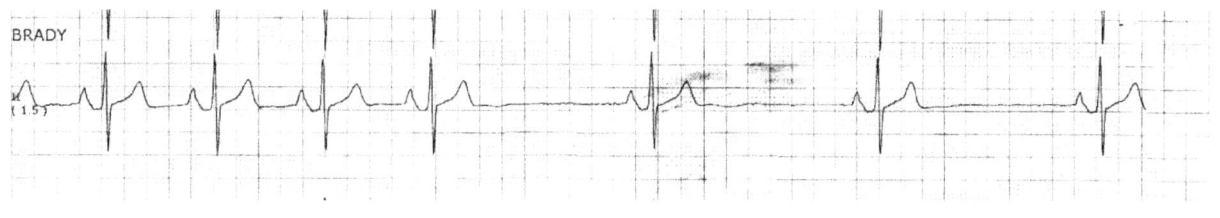

13. _____

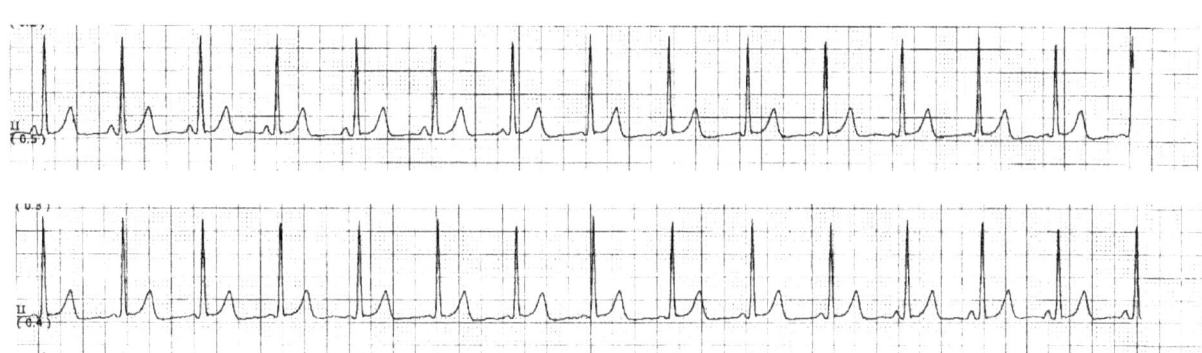

14. _____

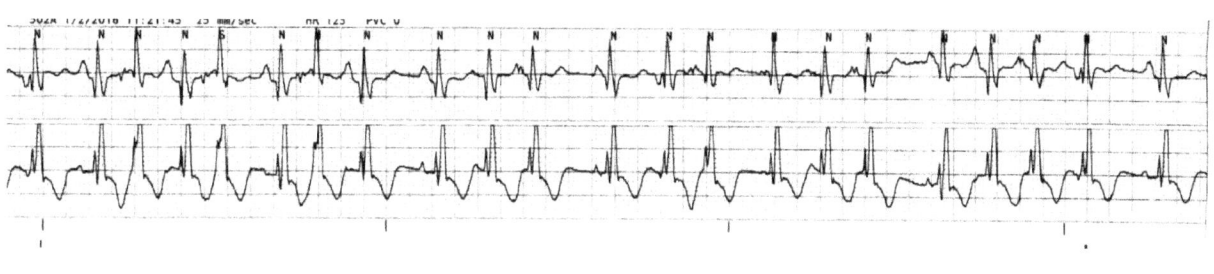

15. _____

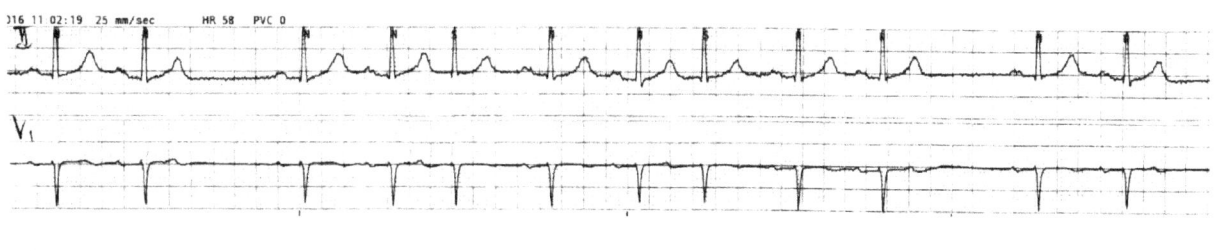

16. _____

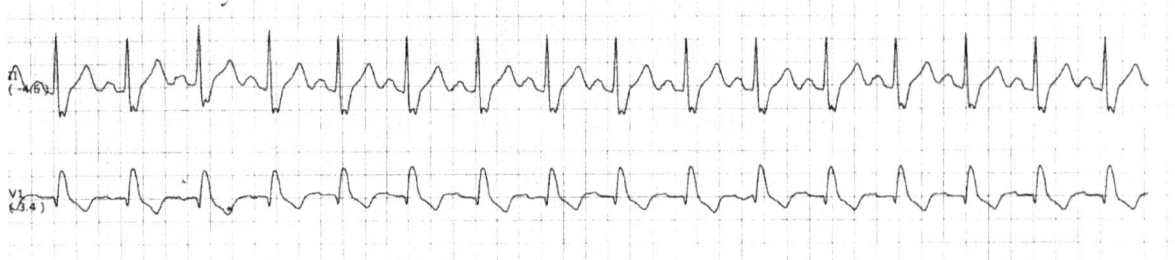

17. _____

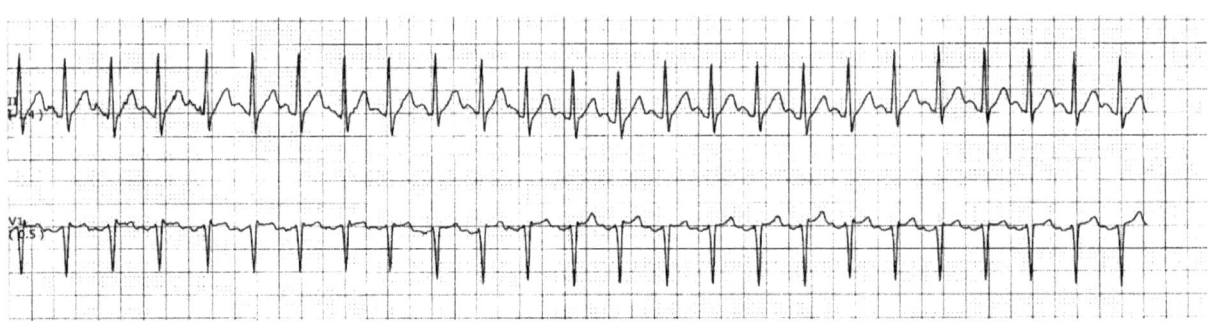

18. _____

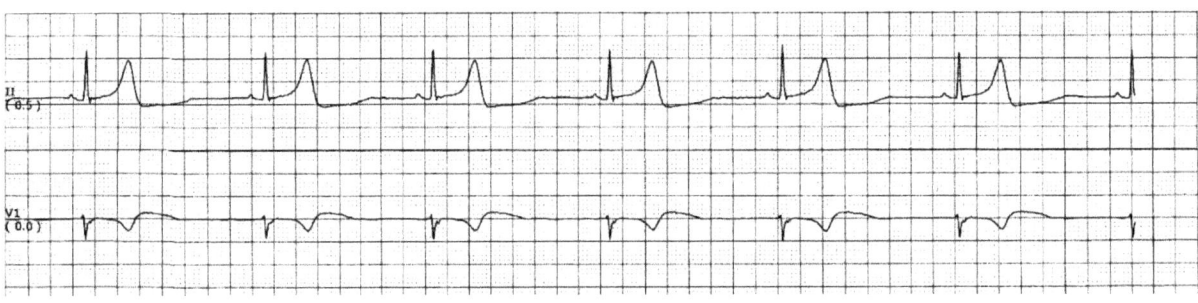

19. _____

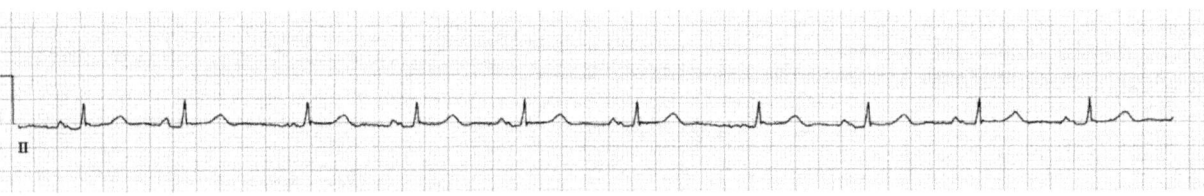

20. _____

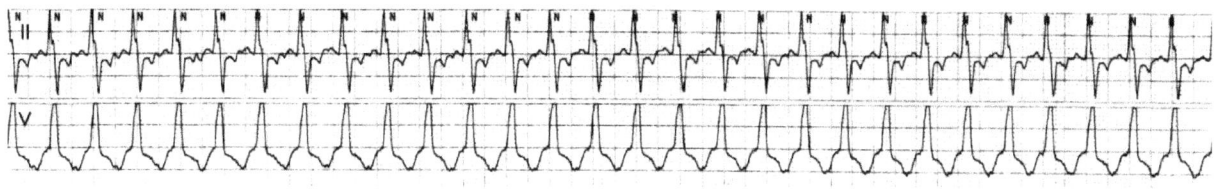

21. _____

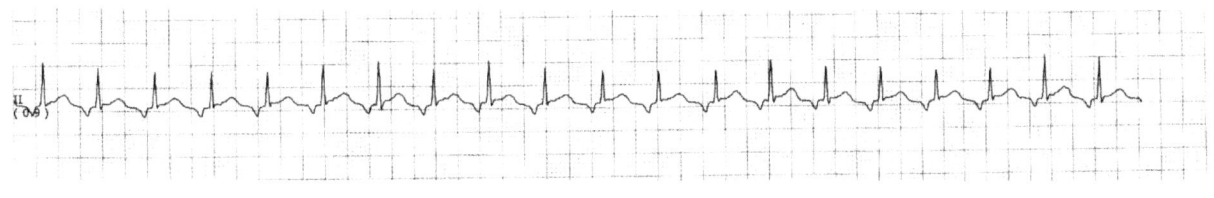

22. _____

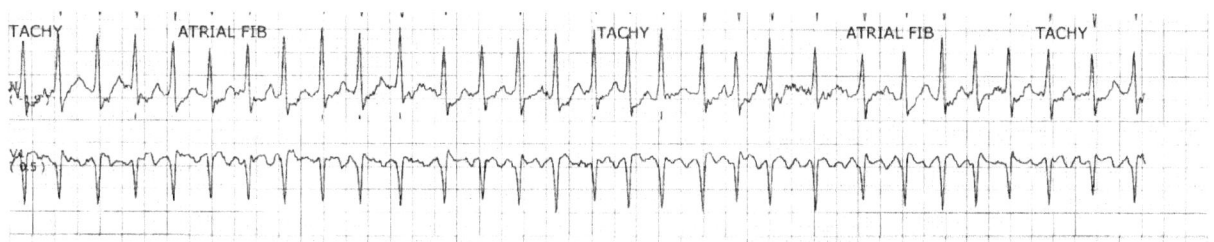

23. _____

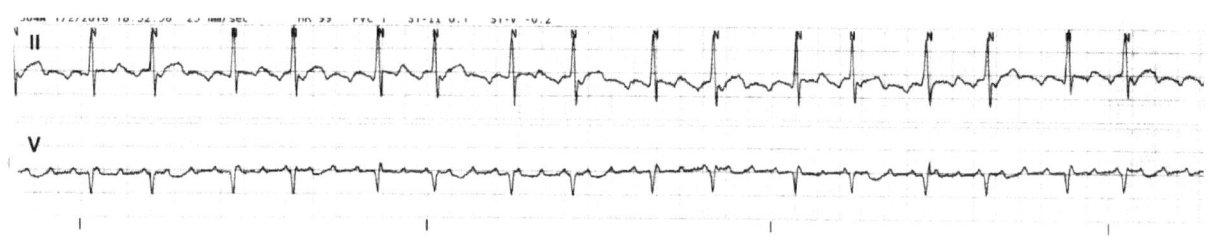

24. _____

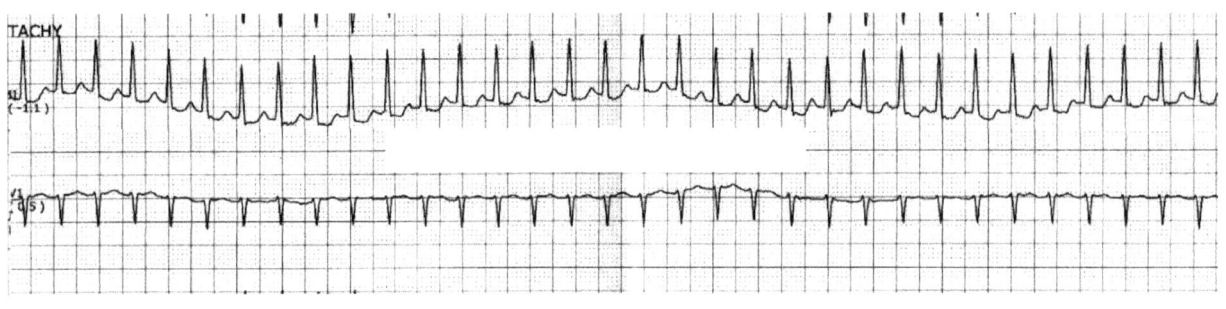

25. _____

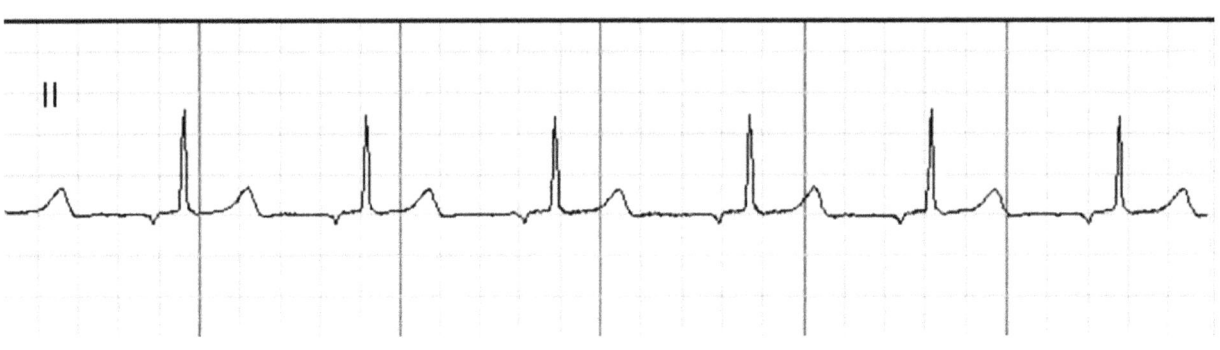

26. _____

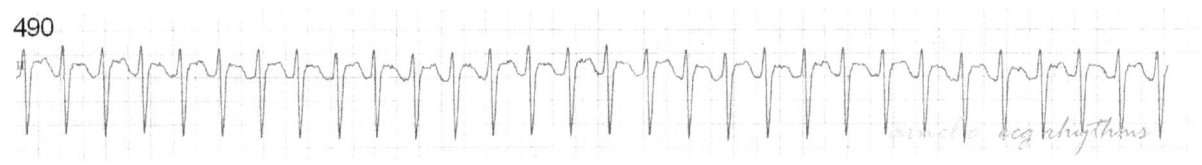

27. _____

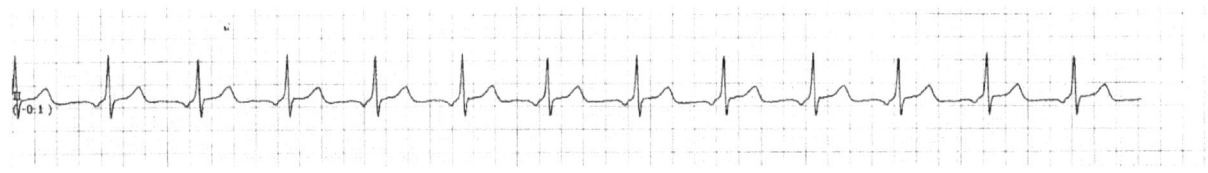

28. _____

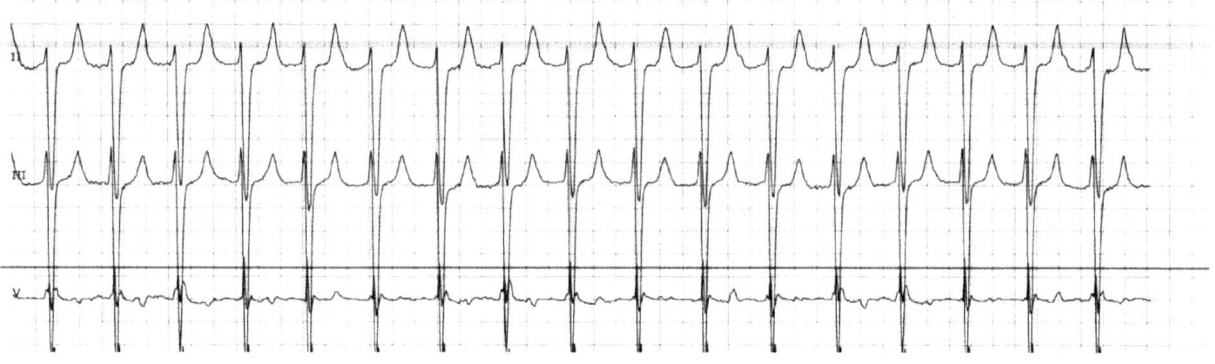

29. _____

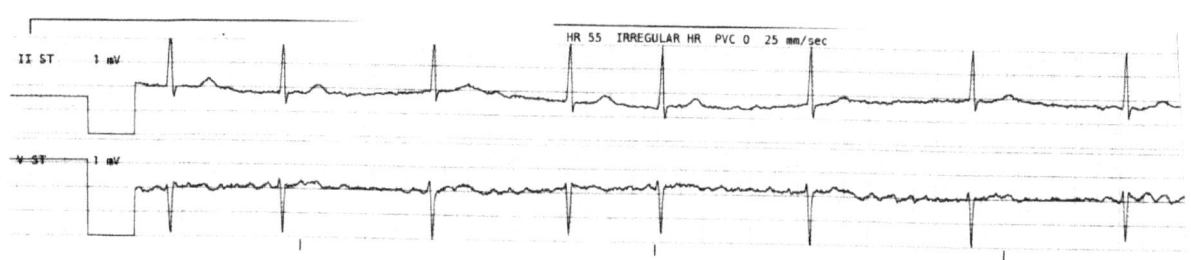

30. _____

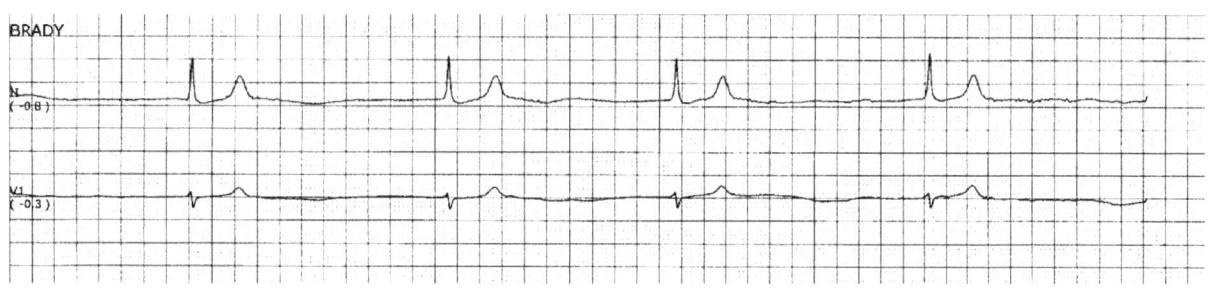

31. _____

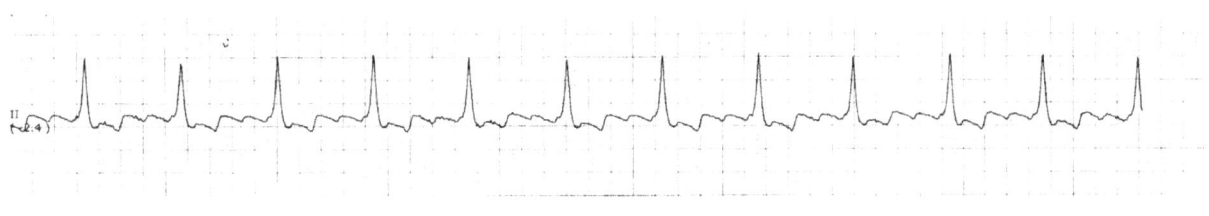

32. _____

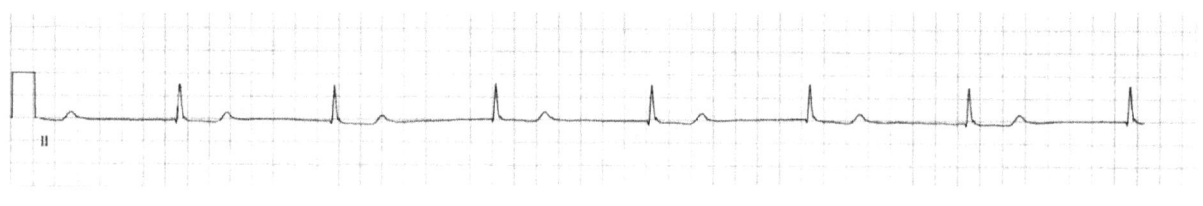

33. _____

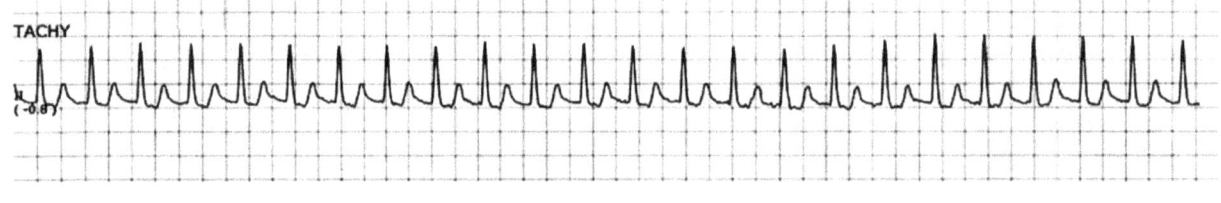

34. _____

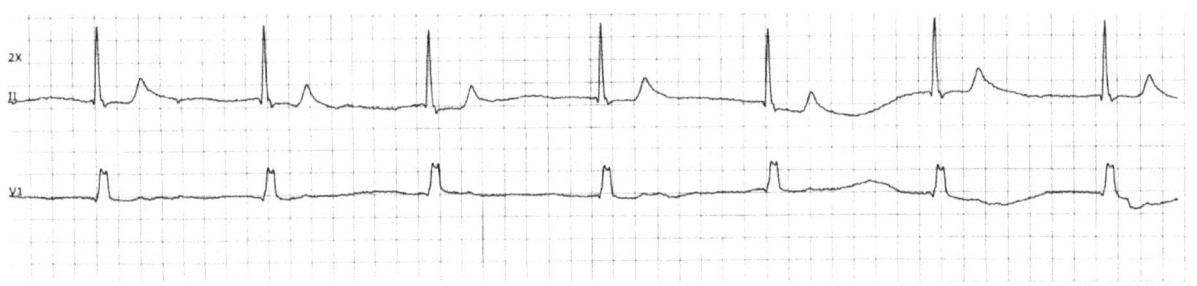

35. _____

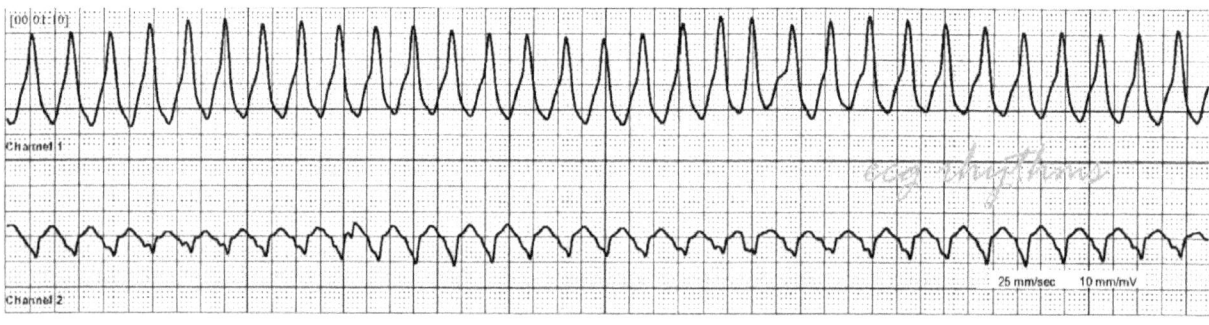

36. _____

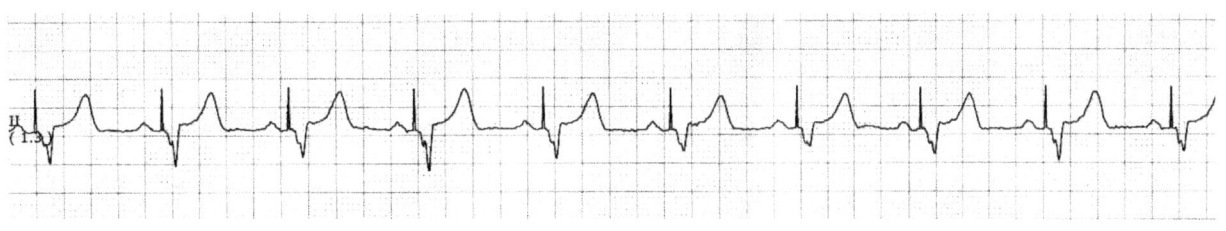

37. _____

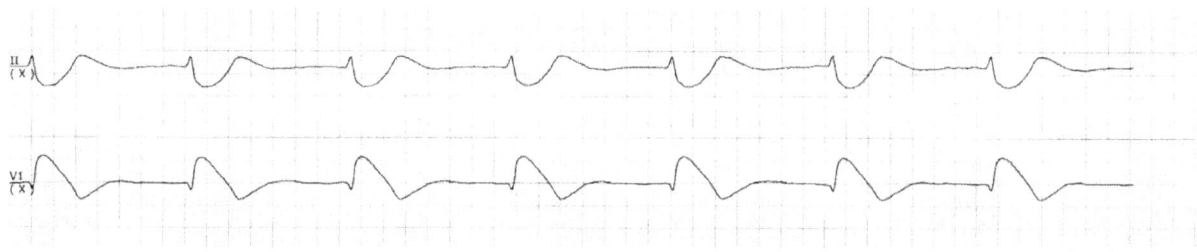

38. _____

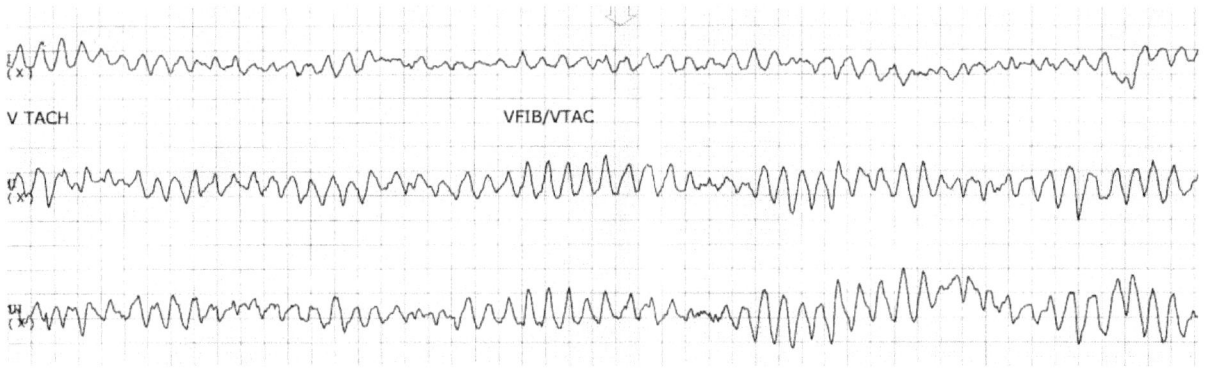

39. _____

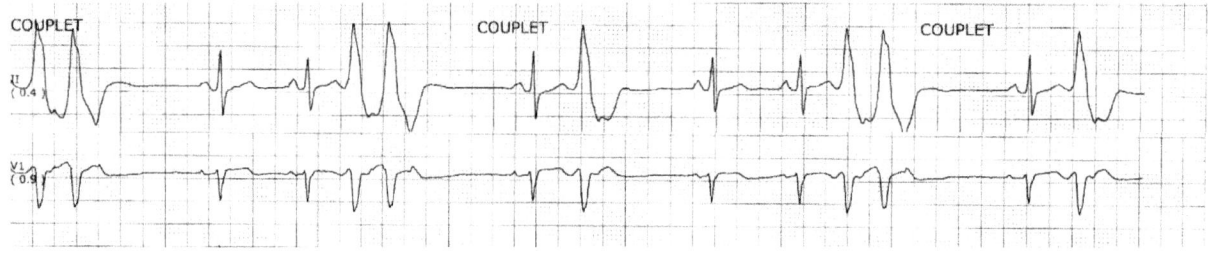

40. _____

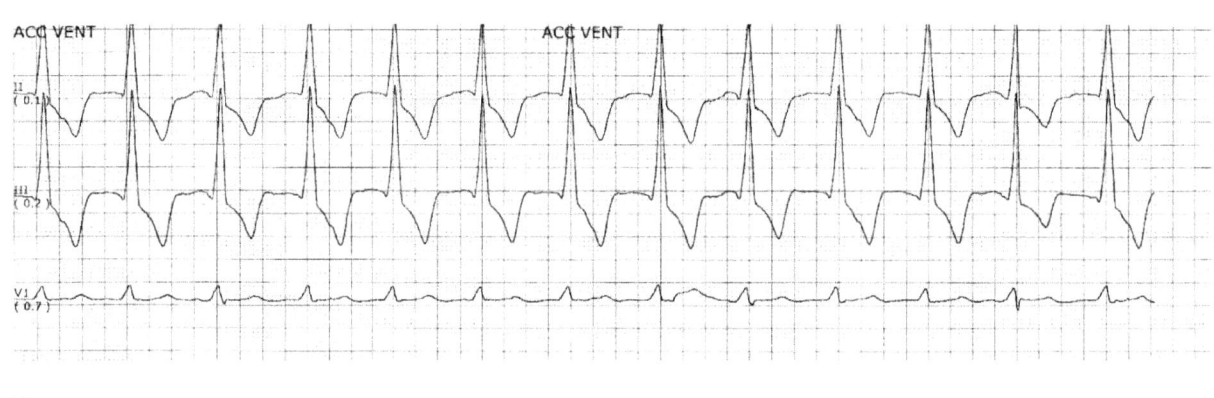

41. _____

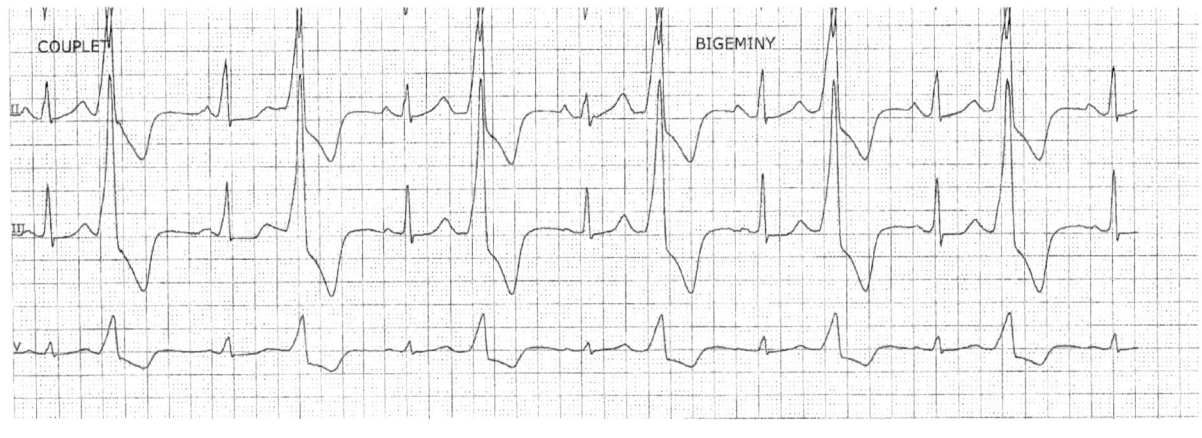

42. _____

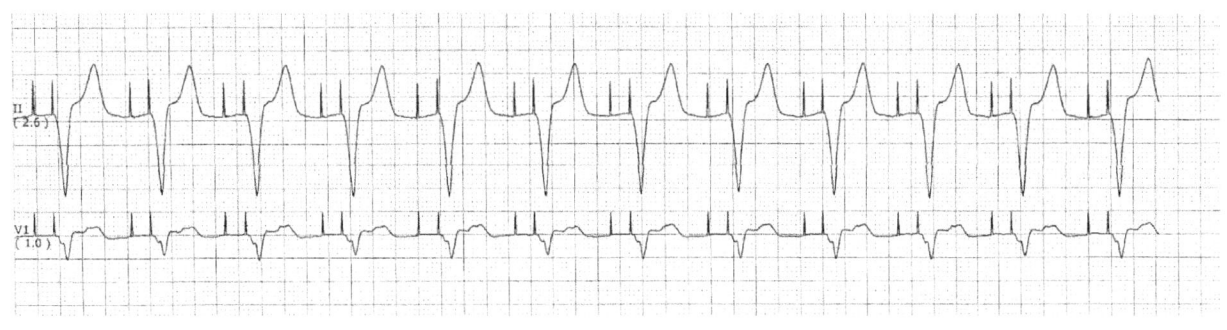

43. _____

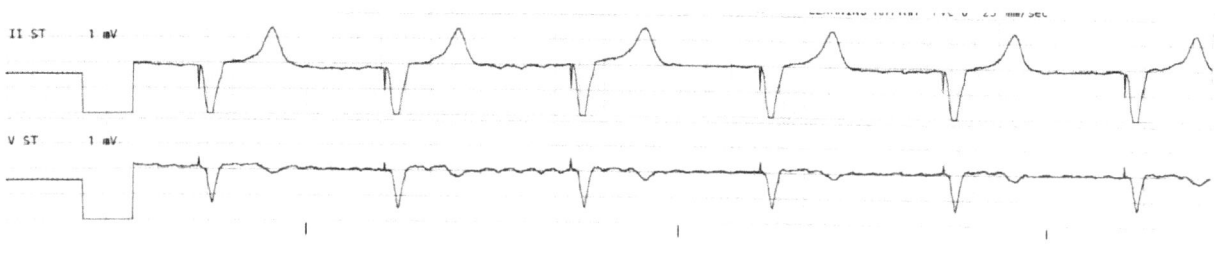

44. _____

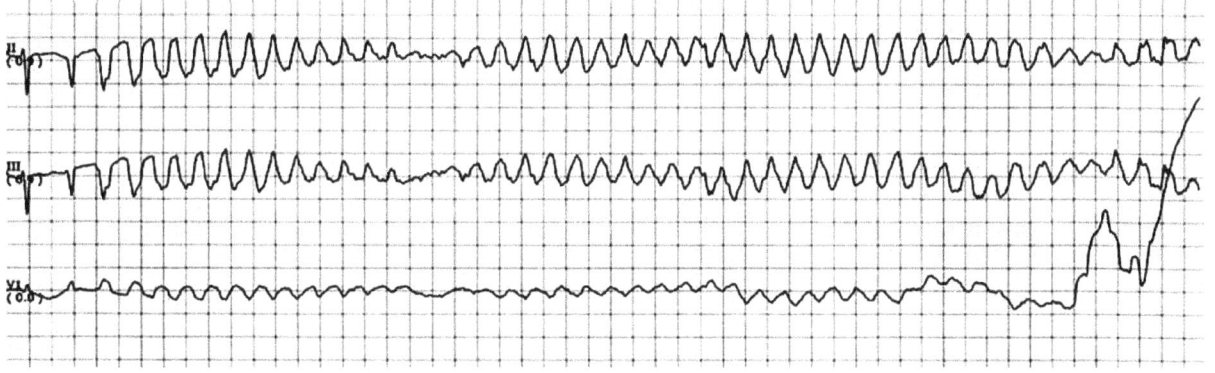

45. _____

71

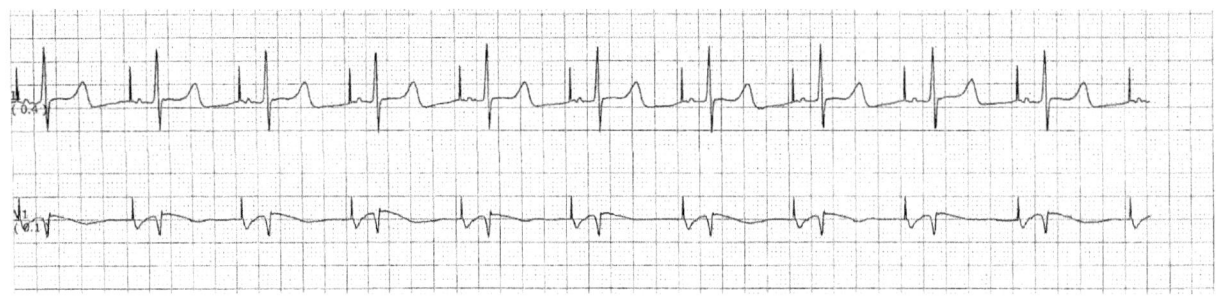

46. _____

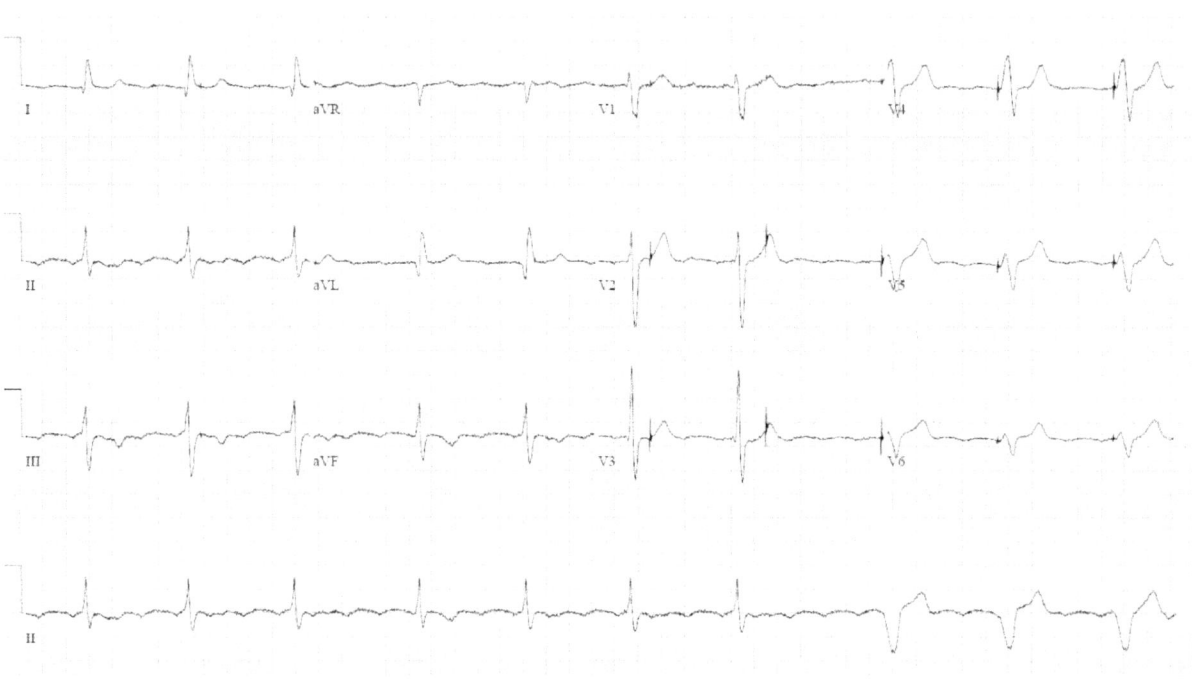

47. _____

QRS changing amplitude
PVC
Short-long-short cycle
QRS Twisting around the isoelectric line
VFIB/VTAC
V TACH
VFIB/VTAC
Heart Rhythms

48. ______________________________

1 2 3 4 5 6 7 8
1 2 3 4 5 6 7 8

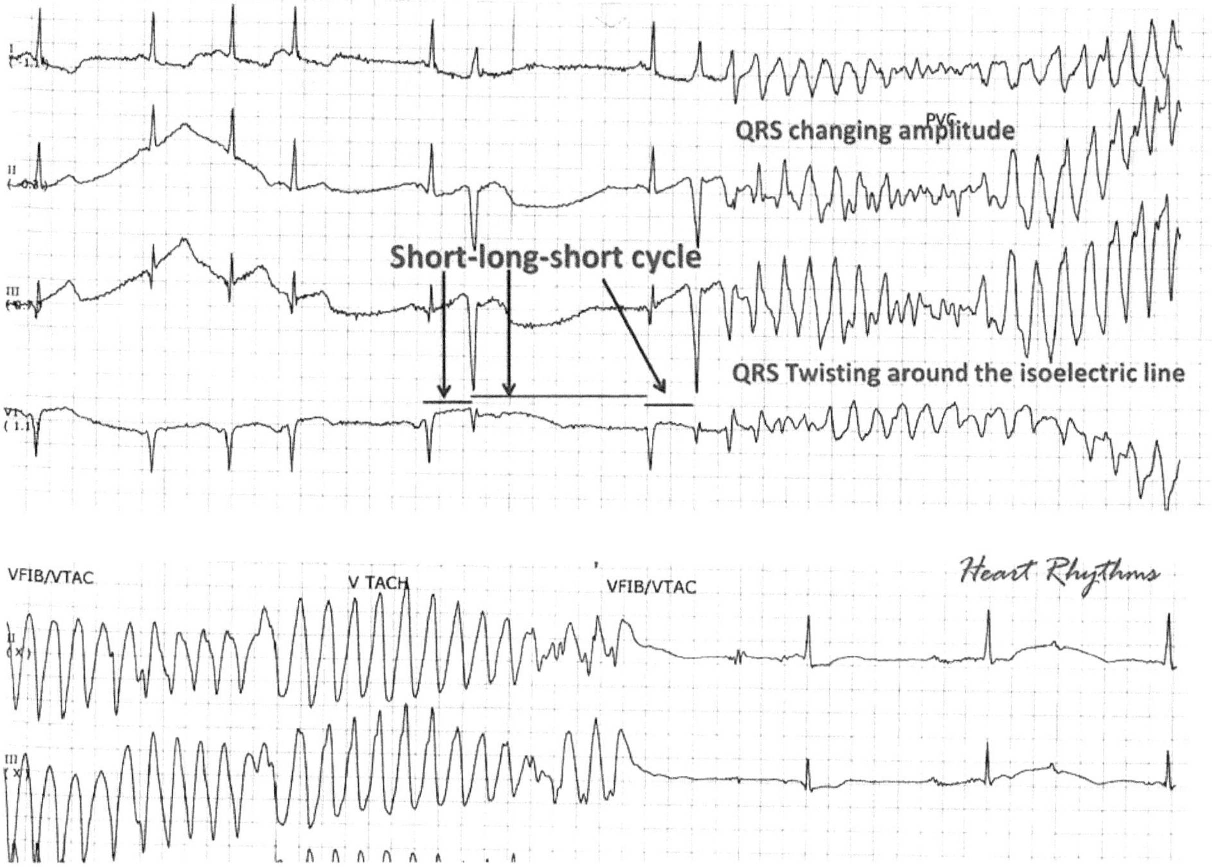

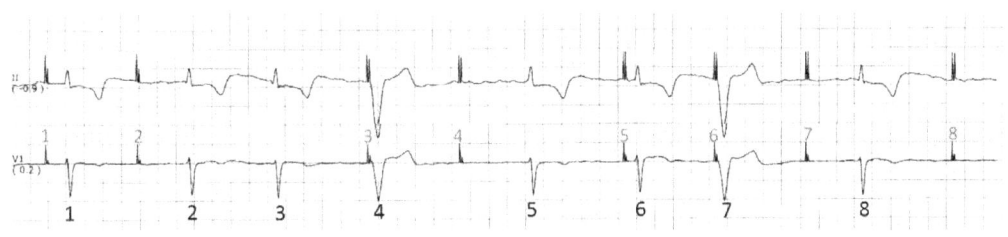

49. ______________________________

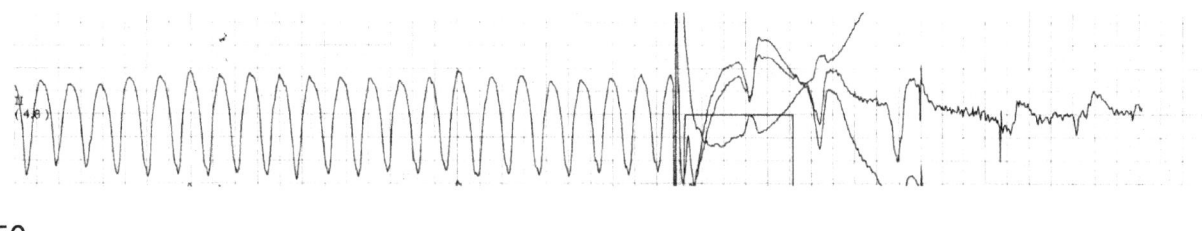

50. ______________________________

Answers:

1. Sinus rhythm, second degree AV block type I (Mobitz I or Wenckebach)

2. Sinus rhythm, second degree AB block type II, bundle branch block

3. Sinus rhythm, first degree AV block, bundle branch block

4. Sinus rhythm, complete heart block or third degree AV block, junctional escape rhythm

5. Paroxysmal AV block or ventricular standstill

6. Second degree AV block 2:1

7. Sinus tachycardia, complete heart block or third degree AV block, idioventricular escape rhythm

8. Sinus tachycardia, advanced or high-degree AV block, bundle branch block

9. Normal sinus rhythm

10. Sinus pause / sinus arrest

11. Sinus arrhythmia

12. Multifocal atrial rhythm / tachycardia

13. Sinoatrial block or sinoatrial exit block

14. Wandering atrial pacemaker

15. Multifocal atrial tachycardia, bundle branch block

16. Sinus rhythm, premature atrial complex (conducted and non-conducted)

17. Sinus rhythm, bundle branch block

18. Sinus tachycardia

19. Sinus bradycardia

20. Sinus arrhythmia

21. Supraventricular tachycardia

22. Junctional tachycardia

23. Atrial fibrillation with rapid ventricular response

24. Atrial flutter with variable block

25. Supraventricular tachycardia

26. Junctional rhythm

27. Supraventricular tachycardia

28. Accelerated junctional rhythm

29. Supraventricular tachycardia

30. Atrial fibrillation with slow ventricular response

31. Junctional rhythm

32. Atrial flutter

33. Junctional rhythm

34. Supraventricular tachycardia

35. Junctional rhythm, bundle branch block

36. Ventricular tachycardia

37. Ventricular pacing, sinus rhythm

38. Idioventricular rhythm

39. Ventricular fibrillation

40. Sinus rhythm, PVC in couplet

41. Accelerated idioventricular rhythm

42. Sinus rhythm, PVC's in bigeminy

43. AV pacing

44. Ventricular or V-pacing

45. Polymorphic ventricular tachycardia

46. Atrial or A-pacing

47. Atrial flutter, ventricular pacing, undersensing with functional non-capture

48. Torsades de Pointes

49. Atrial fibrillation with slow ventricular response in a patient with VVI pacemaker, intermittent failure to capture or loss of capture and intermittent undersensing

50. Ventricular tachycardia terminated with a shock.

Congratulations and goodluck! @Arnel C 2016

References:

Bayes de Luna A. 2011. Clinical Arrhythmology. John Wiley and Sons. UK

Blomström-Lundqvist C, Scheinman M, Aliot E, et al. 2003. ACC/AHA/ESC guidelines for the management of patients with supraventricular arrhythmias*—executive summary: a report of the American college of cardiology/American heart association task force on practice guidelines and the European society of cardiology committee for practice guidelines (writing committee to develop guidelines for the management of patients with supraventricular arrhythmias) Developed in Collaboration with NASPE-Heart Rhythm Society. *J Am Coll Cardiol.* ;42(8):1493-1531.

Bonnow et al. 2014. Braunwald's Heart Disease: A Textbook of Cardiovascular Medicine. 10th Edition. PA.Saunders

Brugada P et al. 1991. A New Approach to the Differential Diagnosis of a Regular Tachycardia With a Wide QRS Complex Circulation 83:1649-1659

Chow AC and Buxton AE. 2006. Defibrillators: All You Wanted to Know. Malden, MA, Blackwell Pub Inc

Das and Zipes. 2012. Electrocardiography of arrhythmias : a comprehensive review. Elsevier PA

Drew B et al. 2010. AHA/ACCF Scientific Statement Prevention of Torsade de Pointes in Hospital Settings. Circulation 121: 1047-1060

Fisch C and Knoebel S. 1992 .Vagaries of Aberrancy. Br Heart J 67:16-24

Fisch C and Knoebel SB. 2000. Electrocardiography of Clinical Arrhythmia. New York. Futura Publishing Co.

Fisch C. 1983. Aberration: seventy five years after Sir Thomas Lewis. Br Heart J; 50: 297 -302

Fisch C., Zipes DP and McHenry PL. 1973. Rate Dependent Aberancy. Circ 48:714-724

Garner JB and Miller JM. 2013. Wide Complex Tachycardia – Ventricular Tachycardia or Not Ventricular Tachycardia, That Remains the Question. Arrhythmia & Electrophysiology Review 2(1):23–29

Goldberger A. 2013. Goldberger's Clinical Electrocardiography : A Simplified Approach 8Ed. Ph Elsevier

Issa Z, Miller J and Zipes D. 2012. Clinical Arrhythmology and Electrophysiology: A Comprehensive Review - A Companion to Braunwald's Heart Disease 2nd Ed. PA Saunders

Kumar UN et al. 2006. The 12L Electrocardiogram in Supraventricular Tachycardia. Cardiology Clinics ;24: 427-437

Malmivuo J and Plonsey R.1995. Bioelectromagnetism - Principles and Applications of Bioelectric and Biomagnetic Fields. Oxford University Press. NY

Marriot HJ. 1998. Pearls and Pitfalls in Electrocardiography (2ed). MA Williams and Wilkins

Miller et al. 2006. The Value of 12-Lead ECG in Wide QRS Tachycardia Cardiology Clinics 24:439-451

Neiger JS and Trohman RG. Differential Diagnosis of Tachycardia with a Typical LBBB Morphology. WJC 3(5):127-134

Prutkim JM. Electrocardiographic and Electrophysiologic Features of type I Atrial Flutter. In:UptoDate: Zimbetbaum PJ and Goldberger AL (Ed)). UpToDate: Waltham, MA 2012

Saoudi N et al.2001. Classification of Atrial Flutter and Regular Atrial Tachycardia According to Electrophysiologic Mechanism and Anatomic Basis: A Statement from Joint Expert Group from the Working Group of Arrhythmias of the European Society of Cardiology and North American Society of Pacing and Electrophysiology. Journal of Cardiovascular Electrophysiology 12: 852-866

Sauer WH. Second Degree AV block: Mobitz I (Wenckebach block): In UpToDate, Gaz LI (Ed), UpToDate, Walthham, MA, 2012

Sousa et al. 2012. The Value of Electrocardiography in the Differential Diagnosis of Wide QRS Complex Tachycardia. Rev Port Cardiol 33:165-173

Stahmer SA and Cowan R. 2006. Tachydysrhythmias. Emergency Medicine Clinics of North America 24:11-40

Surawicz B and Knilans TK. 2008. Chou's Electrocardiography in Clinical Practice. 6th ed. PA. Saunders-Elseiver

Ufberg JW and Clark JS. 2006. Bradyarrhythmias and AV Conduction Blocks. Emergency Clinics of North America ; 24:1-9

Varriale P et al.1992. Multifocal Atrial Arrhythmia-A Frequent Misdiagnosis? A Correlative Study Using the Computerized ECG.Clin. Cardiol. 15,343-346

Wang K.2013. Altas of Electrocardiography. India Jaypee Bros

Wellens HJ. 2001. Ventricular tachycardia: diagnosis of broad QRS complex tachycardia. *Heart* 86:579–585

Index

accelerated idioventricular rhythm 5, 58
Accelerated junctional rhythm 30
Advanced/High-degree AV block 5, 41
Atrial Fibrillation 5, 50
Atrial Flutter 5, 46, 68
Atrial Tachycardia 5, 49, 68
Atrioventricular Block 4, 33
AV junction 8, 32, 44
AV Junctional Rhythms 4, 30
AV node 8, 12, 28, 29, 33, 38, 43, 49, 50, 52
Big box/square method 4, 13
bradycardia 16
Bundle branch block 18
cardiac conduction system 7
ECG paper 6
failure to capture 63, 64, 65
failure to sense 66
First Degree AV Block 4, 12, 33
functional non-capture 66
His Bundle Branch 4, 8
How to compute the rates 13
Idioventricular Rhythm 5, 58
Junctional rhythm 30, 31
Junctional tachycardia 30
Leads 4, 9
loss of capture 64, 65
Mobitz I 5, 35, 68
Mobitz II 5, 22, 38, 41, 42
Monomorphic VT 62
Multifocal Atrial Arrhythmia 4, 24
Multifocal Atrial Rhythm 4, 24
Multifocal Atrial Tachycardia 4, 24
Non-phasic sinus arrhythmia 4, 22
normal sinus rhythm 16
P wave 11, 12, 16, 17, 18, 19, 20, 21, 22, 23, 24, 25, 28, 29, 30, 31, 32, 33, 35, 36, 38, 39, 40, 41, 42, 43, 44, 45, 49, 54, 56, 57, 63, 66
P wave duration 12
P, QRS, T 11
PAC 45

Paced Rhythms 5, 63
Paroxysmal AV block 5, 45
Phasic sinus arrhythmia 4, 21
Polymorphic VT 60
PR interval (PRI) 12, 16
Premature Atrial Complexes 4, 28
Premature Ventricular Complexes 5, 56
Purkinje fibers 4, 7, 8
QRS complex 11, 19, 22, 30, 31, 38, 44, 48, 49, 51, 52, 53, 55, 57, 61, 64, 65, 68
QRS duration 12, 19, 28, 39, 40
QT interval 12
Second Degree AV Block 5, 35
Second degree AVB Type I 5, 35, 37
Second degree AVB Type II 5, 38
Sinoatrial Block 4, 25
Sinoatrial exit block 4, 25, 26
Sinoatrial Node 4, 8
Sinoatrial Rhythms 4, 16
Sinus arrest 4, 27
Sinus Arrhythmia 4, 21, 22
Sinus Bradycardia 4, 19
Sinus Node 4, 8
Sinus Rhythm 4, 16
Sinus Tachycardia 4, 20
Six (6) -second method 4, 15
Small box/square method 4, 13, 14
Supraventricular Tachycardia 5, 52, 67
T wave 11, 12, 29, 30, 33, 36, 56
tachycardia 16
Third Degree AV Block 5, 43
Torsades de Pointes 60, 61
undersensing 64, 65
ventricular fibrillation 62
Ventricular Rhythms 5, 56
ventricular standstill 5, 45
Ventricular Tachycardia 5, 59, 68
Ventriculophasic sinus arrhythmia 4, 22
Wandering Atrial Pacemaker 4, 23
Wenckebach 5, 35, 36, 37, 40, 49, 68

www.ingramcontent.com/pod-product-compliance
Lightning Source LLC
Chambersburg PA
CBHW080625190526
45169CB00009B/3293